"In her latest group therapy textbook, Dr. Brown masterfully develops a unique focus on how best to educate and train group therapists. This is a well written, very important and timely textbook, responding to the expanding utilization of the group therapies."

Molyn Leszcz, *MD, FRCPC, CGP, AGPA-DF, Professor of Psychiatry, University of Toronto; Past-President, the American Group Psychotherapy Association*

"*Teaching Facilitation of Group Therapy* captures the essence and complexity of skills of effective group leadership. It covers both the basics and essential knowledge, skill and characteristics required to run an array of groups. A must read for aspiring group leaders."

Gary M Burlingame, *PhD, CGP, AGPA-DF, APA-F, Professor & Chair, BYU Psychology Department; President, American Group Psychotherapy Association*

"What a treasure to find a book the integrates my two favorite worlds – pedagogy and group psychotherapy. As someone who has taught group courses many times, I was delighted that it both consolidated what I have come to know and unveiled novel content. Both seasoned and brand–new instructors alike will cherish this gift."

Noelle Lefforge, *Ph.D., ABPP., Clinical Associate Professor University of Denver Graduate School of Professional Psychology Associate Dean for Applied Research and Sponsored Programs*

Teaching Facilitation of Group Therapy

Teaching Facilitation of Group Therapy explores an extensive range of topics crucial to effective teaching and practice, and will be a valuable resource for instructors of group therapy.

With an emphasis on evidence-based methodologies, this book describes proven teaching techniques that foster a dynamic learning environment, facilitate group cohesion, and promote meaningful interventions. The author presents ethical considerations including those that relate to using social media in therapeutic practices, equipping readers with the knowledge to leverage its potential while safeguarding client confidentiality and well-being. This resource presents topics including therapeutic factors and effective interventions, the use of the group leader's inner development as a guide for therapeutic alliance and group members' healing, cutting-edge therapeutic AI applications, the role of self-absorption for members and the leader, group dynamics, ethical uses of social media in therapeutic settings, and serves as a comprehensive guide for instructors in the art of teaching group psychotherapy in the modern era.

This is an indispensable resource for educators to elevate their expertise in teaching group psychotherapy and prepare clinicians and students by deepening their understanding of group dynamics, and how to employ effective interventions that promote healing and growth in therapeutic settings.

Nina W. Brown, EdD., is a professor and eminent scholar in the department of Counseling and Human Services at Old Dominion University, a Licensed Professional Counselor, a Nationally Certified Counselor, a Distinguished Fellow in the American Group Psychotherapy Association, and a Fellow in the American Psychological Association.

Teaching Facilitation of Group Therapy

Processes and Applicati

Nina W. Brown

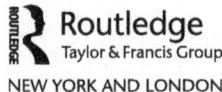

Routledge
Taylor & Francis Group

NEW YORK AND LONDON

Designed cover image: © Getty Images

First published 2024
by Routledge
605 Third Avenue, New York, NY 10158

and by Routledge
4 Park Square, Milton Park, Abingdon, Oxon OX14 4RN

Routledge is an imprint of the Taylor & Francis Group, an informa business

© 2024 Nina W. Brown

Library of Congress Cataloging-in-Publication Data
A catalog record for this title has been requested

ISBN: 978-1-032-36005-8 (hbk)
ISBN: 978-1-032-36004-1 (pbk)
ISBN: 978-1-003-32978-7 (ebk)

DOI: 10.4324/9781003329787

Typeset in Bembo
by Taylor & Francis Books

This book is dedicated to our son Michael (1960–2019) who is forever in our hearts

Contents

Preface

Following are some quotes from the previous book that I wrote on teaching group therapy, *Teaching Group Dynamics: Process and Practice*, published in 1992 (Brown, 1992). These quotes also apply to this current book, as there were and are no books dedicated to assisting instructors how to best present the material that will allow students to become effective clinicians. In the 1992 book I wrote:

> This book was written because current texts on group therapy did not meet my instructional needs. Many are excellent for student purposes but less so for instructional or training purposes.
>
> I wanted a book that presented me with processes for teaching ambiguous concepts central to group dynamics: identifying resistances and knowing what to do after they are identified; helping students grow in self-awareness and knowing or documenting that such growth has taken place. I could accept that much of what I was seeking is subjective in nature, but I did want to have some assurance that the messages were being received.
>
> Numerous books on group therapy cover major topics very well. Issues of group membership, theory, stages of development, and leadership styles may be given differing attention depending on the author, but most group therapy books give adequate information. However, even the best of these did not provide enough information on how best to teach the concepts so as to not lose the complexity and dynamism of the group in actions.

The process that was developed and presented in 1992 has as its foundation the idea that the essence of the therapist is the single most important factor and is emphasized in the 70–15–15 model that is presented in the current book. The idea follows Yalom's emphasis on the development of the group leader's inner self and practice accomplished through "deliberate practice, self-reflection, feedback, and use of empathic and attuned therapeutic relationship" (Yalom, 1995, p. 10). These concepts are used to promote the integration of self-development with presentation of didactic and cognitive material so that students will learn about themselves while learning about group processes and procedures, as well as expanding their knowledge about others in the world.

Another premise is that teaching differs from clinical practice in many ways, but the essential differences are the ethical concerns, including that students are not group members either voluntary or involuntary, the didactic and cognitive concerns that there is specific knowledge about the technical aspects of group that promote effectiveness for group members learning and change, and the many intangibles that group leaders will encounter but are difficult to adequately define and describe. The instructor of the group therapy course has to be mindful of these differences when organizing and directing the class, as well as the importance of teaching the clinical aspects of group therapy.

My hope is that the material presented in this book will help guide instructors in their teaching of group therapy and assist them to develop their own unique instructional style that will incorporate the essentials for becoming an effective group leader.

References

Brown, N. (1992). *Teaching Group Dynamics: Process and Practice*. Westport, CT: Praeger.

Yalom, I. (1995). *The Theory and Practice of Group Psychotherapy*. New York: Basic Books.

Acknowledgments

I want to acknowledge the contributions that many have made to the production of this book. The information I received from attending conferences of the American Group Psychotherapy Association (AHPA) and from experienced clinicians was invaluable in deciding what entering group therapists will find most helpful in their future practices. The experts I had opportunities to interact with at the Society for Group Psychology and Group Psychotherapy (APA Division 49) also added to my knowledge and understanding of group therapy.

I want to especially thank Gary Burlingame (current president of AGPA), who had always been supportive; Noelle Lefforge current president of the Society (APA), a valued colleague; and Molyn Lesczc, former president of AGPA, who was always encouraging and a role model. Colleagues at Old Dominion University who made contributions to my understanding of cybersecurity and were willing to answer questions were Doug Streit, the Executive Director of IT Security and Planning, and Roderick Graham, from the Department of Sociology. There are many other professionals and colleagues who deserve thanks for their dissemination of clinical information that helped with writing this book.

Finally, many thanks to Amanda Savage, my editor, who was always willing to answer my questions and did so promptly.

1 Teaching Group Therapy Components and Strategies

C felt panic because their teaching assignment for the next year is the entry-level course on group therapy. C. was feeling disconcerted and having chaotic thoughts because not only was this a new course, but it was not clear how to present the complex concepts about group therapy to ensure learning for the students. Although C. also had a private practice that was composed of individual clients, they had not facilitated a group since their doctoral studies a few years ago. Like most first-time teachers for group therapy C. realized that they were going to have to rely on using how they were taught to teach this assigned class. The most troubling thoughts were about what to teach, how to teach it, and how to know if what was planned would be effective.

R. was a tenured professor who had taught group therapy for several years but had become increasingly less satisfied with what and how they were teaching. R. used a textbook that was highly respected by others who taught group therapy, had refined their teaching techniques to incorporate new findings about group therapy, and other such actions, but was not convinced that what they were doing was the best way to help students learn. If asked what did not seem effective, R. would probably respond that students did not seem to understand how to use the resources of the group to help individual group members (but seemed to insist on working with individual members in the group setting), nor how to identify and intervene for some group intangibles, and were uncomfortable with not having specific techniques that were always effective as interventions.

These are two common examples of what many instructors of group therapy face when trying to organize a course. They are unsure how to organize the learning so that the complexity for group leaders is understood as well as the information about effective interventions. This is made even more complex as neither the instructor nor the students know what problems, concerns, conditions, or even the target audiences for their groups in the future. This book is intended to provide instructors with information and evidence-based strategies for teaching group therapy regardless of the type of group and for the variety of members and their needs that students may encounter.

A search of publishers showed that there are no books on teaching group therapy other than the previous one published in 1992 (Brown, 1992).

DOI: 10.4324/9781003329787-1

Group therapy is growing as a treatment for many different issues, problems, and concerns, and it is more than just doing individual therapy in a group setting. Group therapy has a unique knowledge and technique base and there are many intangibles that call for considerable self-understanding and awareness on the part of the group leader, and these are difficult to describe and to teach. For example, resistance is a concept that can be somewhat defined, but the definition does not convey how to recognize members' or the group's resistance, nor does it suggest what could be effective interventions. The primary focus for the book is on teaching and included are teaching group therapy concepts, techniques and facilitation strategies based on a proposed 70–15–15 teaching-learning model that emphasizes the psychological, cognitive, and emotional development of the group leader.

The 70–15–15 Group Leadership/Teaching Model

The teaching model is based on the understanding that the most important components for effective group leadership are the leader and their expertise (Yalom & Leszcz, 2021), and that there are both art and science components for what is to be taught. Other factors are important, but it is important to place the emphasis for teaching group therapy on the most important component, and since most of what comprises this component are the self-knowledge, self-awareness and self-understanding of the group leader, the instructors who have to teach group leadership will want to make this component the emphasis and focus of their teaching. This book highlights the group leader's self-development and its impact on the group's progress and process as well as its influences on group members' healing, growth and development, and how to is to incorporate this most important component into the learning experiences for the course as many of the aspects are complex and intangible.

This 70 percent (the leader's inner developed therapeutic self), 15 percent (information about group dynamics and factors), and 15 percent (learned techniques and strategies) model for teaching and learning is based on three main premises: first, the development of the inner self of the group leader is the most important component for effective group facilitation, second is learning the components of the unique knowledge base for group therapy, and third that there are strategies and techniques that can be learned and are shown to promote growth, development and healing for group members. While it is easy for the knowledge and strategies to be conceptualized and presented, it is not easy to describe and illustrate the importance of the therapeutic inner self of the group leader. The therapeutic inner self of the group leader is defined as being the most important component for successful group therapy as it being the group leader's self-understanding that influences and impact their understanding of the group members and of the group as a whole, and this self-understanding promotes the understanding of the needs of group members as well as those of the group. It is for these reasons that considerable attention is given to helping group leaders in training to become self-reflective.

The Developed Inner Therapeutic Self (70%)

It may be helpful to first briefly describe what is meant by the therapeutic inner self (70%) which is covered more extensively in Chapter 3. The *therapeutic inner self* is conceptualized as the developed inner self, personal attributes, and understanding of one's life experiences, the group leader's self-perception, extent of undeveloped narcissism, psychological boundary strength, influences of the unconscious and associations with counter-transference, awareness of emotional experiencing, and the ability to engage in self-reflection. A *developed inner therapeutic self* refers to having examined and freely chosen values, beliefs, attitudes as well as an awareness of their influences on behaviors and other actions. These play major roles in establishing a therapeutic relationship with group members, under-standing the impact of their life experiences on their present selves, and can be used as guides for when and how to intervene. *Personal attributes* such as warmth, caring, tolerance, and positive regard have been shown to be essential for establishing a trusting and safe group climate but are more related to the personal attributes of the group leader than to anything else. These cannot be taught or practiced, they are inner characteristics that are an essential part of the person. What can be taught and learned are the importance and impact these have for group members, but not how to attain them. The importance of the group leader's *life experiences* for understanding the group and its members, and for knowing how and when to intervene cannot be overly estimated. Experiences such as family of origin experiences especially unresolved issues emanating from the family, unfinished business from other relationships, the past and cultural and social environment are samples of life experiences that may be influential for the group leader as well as bases for understanding group members. Just as with group members, the group leader's perceptions of their self-worth, self-esteem, self- acceptance are an integral part of them and can play a role in the attitudes and actions they bring to leading groups. These perceptions can affect how they relate to group members, their choices for how and when to intervene, management of conflict and problem behaviors and other important group concerns. There is also the possibility of the leader projecting their self-perceptions onto group members and by doing so, affect members' behaviors.

The extent of the leader's *undeveloped narcissism and developed healthy adult narcissism* play an integral part in the facilitation of the groups. Aspects of these can unconsciously affect the choices of interventions, emotional pre-sence, and most of all how they relate to group members. Undeveloped narcissistic behaviors and attitudes such as grandiosity, impoverished ego, entitlement, exploitation, lack of empathy, attention and admiration needs, envy, and extensions of self can have negative effects on the group and its members. The extent of development for healthy adult narcissism of empathy, wisdom, an appropriate sense of humor, zest, and appreciation of beauty and wonder can have positive effects. Both undeveloped and healthy adult narcissism are presented in Chapter 6.

The importance of the group leader's *psychological boundary strength* cannot be overly estimated. Their psychological boundary strength contributes to their being able to withstand projections, resist projective identifications and the unconscious impact of emotional contagion. In addition, they can provide a model for group members for how to resist manipulation, coercion, and seduction to do things they do not want to do or are not in their best interests.

Also important is the awareness of how and when they are experiencing the possibility of *unconscious* factors such as transference and counter-transference as well as unresolved issues from past experiences. These factors seem to be present for everyone but are not always recognized as such and for the group leader can play a role for their group leadership. A here and now awareness of their *emotional experiencing* is also important for the group leader's understanding of what the group may be signaling but not verba-lizing as needs and fears, allows them to know when they are acting as the container for members' distressing feelings, and can allow them to model constructive management of intense and uncomfortable feelings. *Self-reflection* is highly encouraged for group leader to both learn more about themselves and their relationships to the group and the members, as a means of monitoring countertransference, and to increase understanding of the unspoken needs and feelings for the group. Reflecting on what was experienced during sessions can help identify what might have been missed, deepen the understanding of how or if interventions worked, and other positive outcomes for leadership. Prompts, activities, and vignettes are presented throughout the book to help integrate the self-development of the therapeutic inner self.

Group Therapy Knowledge Factors (15%)

Central to leading effective therapy groups are some basic knowledge about how groups function, management of group difficulties and concerns, and basic knowledge of some ethical and cultural factors that will affect the group members and the group. Basic knowledge factors include leadership skills, stages of group development, group therapeutic factors, managing intangi-bles, members' diagnoses and conditions, difficulty behaviors, ethics, culture and diversity, and some best practices from current professional literature. Additional information about group stages is presented in Chapter 5.

Fundamental *leadership skills* will include how to organize a group, establish trust and safety, build the therapeutic alliance, identify and repair empathic failures, and manage emotional intensity. While it may appear that these are skills that can be taught and learned it is helpful to remember that embedded in all of these skills will be the developed therapeutic inner self of the group leader. Yes, these can be described, but to be most effective they also have to have the group leader's understanding of their selves. Chapters 6–8 elaborate on these skills.

Group leaders will find it helpful to know and understand the *stages of group development* as these can aid in knowing what the group members can want and need throughout the life span of the group, provide clues for effective interventions, and to reduce some of the ambiguity and uncertainty about expectations. Stages of group development are not fixed except for the beginning stage, as all groups have to begin somewhere, and the ending stage, as all groups will end (or at least members will end the group experience). There are other stages that can contribute to the group leader's understanding of the particular group and its members and provide suggestions for how best to proceed.

Yalom and Leszcz (2021) continue to provide evidence for the existence of 11 *group therapeutic factors* and how these contribute to the growth, development and healing for group members. These factors can be most effectively used as means to understand and foster interpersonal relationships, provide resources that help group members such as universality, hope and altruism, and create a therapeutic environment so that members can better focus on their concerns.

There is no question that *ethics* are critical components for group therapy. All mental health professional organizations have ethical standards but most of these are not specifically applied to group therapy with the exception of the American Group Psychotherapy Association and the International Board of Certified Group Psychotherapists that publishes ethical guidelines for group therapists (AGPA & IBCGP, 2002). This distinction can be important as there can be some unique situations for groups and it is essential that group leaders remain aware of these and how they can affect the group, its members and the leader's professional lives. Examples of unique group ethical considerations are social media posting by group members, confidentiality and privacy and technology.

It is well established that *culture and diversity* play a significant role for the leader and group members, and it is important to understand what impact these have on a particular group and its members. Culture and diversity are complex concepts, and it should be recognized that while generalities may apply to group members, even group members from the same cultural environment can differ in significant ways and the group leader cannot rely on their understanding about a particular culture or of the diversity of group members as fixed traits and must realize that there are individual differences that can apply to their group members. More information about ethics and culture and diversity is presented in Chapter 5.

Considerable findings have and continue to emerge about *members' clinical factors* such as their diagnoses, conditions, and the influences of life experiences. It is most helpful when group leaders stay current with these findings and can use them to better understand the group members' behaviors, attitudes, and actions.

Among the many tasks for the group leader will be *managing difficult member behaviors* so as to not cause a therapeutic rupture and for the benefit of the group as a whole. Behaviors such as monopolizing, storytelling, withdrawal, conflict, and the like can negatively affect the group, and group leaders have to find ways to effectively address the behaviors to promote insight for the member and for the group without blame or criticism. Suggestions to help identify and manage difficult behaviors can be found in Chapter 9.

The advanced skills of *recognizing group process and providing group process commentary* are not easy to describe or understand as these are also intangibles that cannot be readily observed. However, these skills are essential for intervening to help the group to understand what they collectively but in different ways are doing, avoiding, denying and the like. Guides for these advanced skills are presented in Chapter 6.

Group Techniques and Strategies (15%)

There will be a major focus throughout the book on techniques and strategies that are common for all types of groups including clinical, manualized, psychotherapeutic, psychoeducational and support groups. This focus will help to prepare group leaders for a variety of groups to help group leaders understand how and what to do that is effective for the groups as well as for the individual group members. Major topics include planning, treatment planning, the therapeutic alliance, establishing trust and safety, facilitating member to member interactions, interventions such as blocking and encouraging, empathic responding, the importance of empathic responding and identification of empathic failures and repair, fostering the emergence of group therapeutic factors, encouraging and facilitation the expression of feelings, when and how to intervene, managing group intangibles, the corrective emotional experience, and building group cohesion.

Planning the group aids in maintaining a focus on the primary goal and objectives as well as for assessment of effectiveness. Chapters 2 and 4 provide specific information relative to planning and assessment. *Treatment* planning involves the selection of techniques and strategies to guide growth, development, understanding and healing. Additional information can be found in Chapters 4 and 5. *Building a therapeutic alliance* can be critical for the success of the group where the group members can feel safe and trusting enough to let their real selves be seen. Techniques and strategies for building are discussed in Chapters 3 and 7. *Establishing trust and safety* takes a lot of skill as group members may not be open to putting their trust in another person. Also included in the building process are the leader's skills at reducing ambiguity and uncertainty, promotion of inclusion, and addressing fears. Guides for these tasks are presented in Chapters 4 and 7. Facilitative strategies to *guide member to member interactions, and interpersonal feedback* help to produce a healing group climate where members learn to use the resources of the group to aid the individual members. Some strategies for accomplishing these tasks are in Chapter 8. Critical leader tasks and skills are *empathic responding, identification of empathic failures and repair* as basic for establishing the therapeutic alliance, repairing therapeutic ruptures, and encouraging members in self-exploration that may be painful at times. These topics are presented in Chapters 8 and 9. Group leaders will find it helpful to encourage and foster the *emergence of group therapeutic factors* to encourage and support group members as guides for getting better, overcoming obstacles, and in developing better ways to behave and relate. Chapter 6 presents more information about this topic. *Encouraging and supporting the expression of feelings with interpersonal feedback* can be very helpful for group members and the group leader can guide them through this process. Information to aid in guiding members is in Chapter 6. Central to facilitation of the group is knowing *when and how to intervene* especially for difficult group member behaviors and difficult group events such as microaggressions. Several chapters provide guides for the group leader and are primarily found in Chapters 7–9. Learning to *identify and manage group intangibles* such as transference, resistance, projections, and projective identification enhances the effectiveness of the group leader and contributes to their understanding of how and when to intervene. These intangibles cannot be easily described or observed, and it is mainly through the group leader's personal development that they are able to tap into this rich resource for the group's benefit. Chapter 10 presents more detail about these intangibles. Other essential and critical group leader tasks are to *provide corrective emotional experiences and to build group cohesion* and more specific information can also be found in Chapter 10.

Layers of the Teaching Group Therapy Model

The layers for the model are foundational, primer, and acquired learning. The foundational layer is conceptualized as the basic and fundamental self of the group leader. Components for this layer include the family of origin experiences and continuing issues, the unconscious, past experiences especially those that carry unfinished business, personality, undeveloped narcissism and psychological boundary strength. All of these are interrelated and complex, affecting the person without their awareness, which can lead to countertransference and ineffective interventions.

The primer layer encompasses the learned behaviors and attitudes that were internalized as the result of life experiences, values from family and the culture, social convention, and other aspects of self that affected the growth and development for the person. Some of these are in their conscious awareness, but most are acted upon as a part of the person. Many of the group leader's therapeutic attributes, such as tolerance, caring, and concern, reside in this layer.

The final layer is acquired knowledge: generally that which is specifically taught and learned, although there may be some components that were internalized from experiences from the other two layers. Examples of acquired knowledge include communication skills, interpersonal relating style, and problem solving.

These three layers can also be applied to the teaching model. The foundational layer can be conceptualized as using the various learning and psychological theories can be used as the framework for understanding individuals and for the self which can lead to better understanding of group members and how they can to be as they are in the group. The primer layer is how the instructor incorporates and encourages self-reflection, self-exploration, and self-understanding so as to better understand the behaviors and attitudes of group members.

The third layer is developing group facilitation skills, learning how to tune into group dynamics, fundamental communication skills that enhance establishing meaningful connections for and to group members, and other valuable therapeutic skills. Both individual characteristics and group characteristics interact to produce group dynamics which can then be used to better understand and use the resources of the group to help individual group members.

Intangibles are significant group factors and dynamics that can be defined and maybe even described, but they are not seen and, although they affect both the individual group members and the group leader, the definitions and descriptions are not sufficient for understanding. Intangibles like transference and some therapeutic factors are better understood when they emerge and are identified in the moment.

The layers are described separately, as are the components, but they do not usually appear as separate and discrete entities. They appear without awareness, can be embedded in other dynamics, and can be difficult to sort out and identify. This is where the art aspect of teaching group dynamics is most helpful to the instructor.

The layers metaphor is intended to serve as an overview of the complexity for teaching group facilitation, group leaders, group processes, and group members. It is also being used to suggest an order and sequence for building course content that takes into account many intangibles and their contributions such as an understanding of the self of the group leader and of group members, the structural framework of the group and of sessions the techniques and strategies for engaging and guiding group members, and addressing individual and group related problems, issues and concerns. Let's imagine that there are layers to what needs to be taught but that no layer is clearly distinct from the other layers and there are places where one or more previous layers come into play. This is similar to group therapy where invisible forces such as the unconscious or unfinished business are contributing without awareness and only if their presence is understood by the group leader can they be used for interventions, growth, and healing. In therapy, the group and members move between layers, can regress to earlier layers or layers, and can build on previous layers. Even when the layers and forces are understood by the course instructor there is still the added complication of what to teach, when to initiate it, and how to teach it. Much like group dynamics, group forces, therapeutic factors, and other group processes, knowing what they are can be described but the description does not bring understanding or recognition of when they emerge which is the greater challenge for trying to formulate how best to teach about them.

Teaching Layers

What follows conceptualizes teaching group leadership in layers much like those in the metaphor. Those teaching layers are the foundation, previous formal and informal learning experiences, group-level understandings, meanings for intangibles and enhancements. Throughout all of the layers, the underlying and primary focus is on the group leader's therapeutic self, the 70 percent in the teaching model. What follows is a brief description for each layer.

Foundation

This is the primary layer on which the other layers are built. This is the basic layer of the self of the group leader and group members that itself is multifaceted and has multiple layers many of which are invisible, unknown to oneself and not seen by others, and parts that are known to oneself but hidden from others. These significantly affect the beliefs, attitudes and actions for both the leader and members and the course instructor does not know what these are but must try to guide the leaders in training to better understand these for themselves. While the self-understanding is foundational, it is also in continual development of understanding and also serves as a means for some of the understanding of others.

Previous Learning

This is the layer where previous formal and informal learning experiences are accessed and used as building blocks for more advanced understanding and uses. This layer uses other formal learning as the basis for introducing more advanced concepts and skills. An example can be the use of learning for individual therapy as it applies to group therapy. This layer also incorporates previous experiences and shows how these can apply to being a group leader and for understanding group members and is more easily conceptualized as unfinished business from other experiences and relationships, and possible transference and countertransference. This layer incorporates individualized learning for leaders and members about relationships, their value and worth, feelings, and how their thoughts, feelings, and ideas have shaped their selves.

Group-Level Understandings

This is a very complex layer where the previous layers are used to better tune into group dynamics, effective communication skills, developing a therapeutic alliance, how and when to effectively intervene, and other valuable group therapeutic skills. Both individual and group characteristics interact to produce group dynamics which can be useful to the group leader to both understand the needs for individual group members and for the group as a whole. This understanding allows the group leader to better use the resources of the group to help individual group members.

Meanings

All of the previous layers are used to produce meanings and understandings for many of the intangibles in group therapy. Intangibles such as transference, resistance, emergence of difficult and problematic group member behaviors, therapeutic factors and their emergence, interventions for conflicts, and other such intangibles that are always present, not always in the awareness, but that can make significant contributions to the group and its members.

This metaphor and descriptions are the framework for the instructional model, methods, and suggestions presented to teach group therapy leadership. Presented next are the decisions about major learning components for a course, developing measurable goals and objectives, and possible teaching-learning strategies. These will be the same for courses of all lengths and durations, and for in-person or virtual and all are intended to incorporate the 70–15–15 group leadership/teaching model. Adjustments for prevailing course circumstances can be easily made with the proposed course organization. It is very helpful for group instructors to intentionally plan for what is to be taught, the sequence for the materials, and select the strategies in advance of the course. Just as in group therapy, some student needs may not be determined in advance and will emerge during the course, and instructors must have the same flexibility as group leaders for adjusting the course requirements.

Perceptual Shifts

There are some perceptual shifts that are needed to better understand how group therapy differs from other therapies and why group leaders will find it helpful to better understand group dynamics as a means for helping the individual members. The major perceptual shifts include the following.

- Focus on the group as a whole instead of only individual group members to make best use of the resources of the group to help individual group members.
- Observe and understand interactions among and between members, and how these may be reflective of transference, of how they behave and related in interpersonal interactions outside of group session.
- Identify similarities among members that can be meaningful and help them to establish connections.
- Effective use of group dynamics to understand what the group as a whole is telling the leader that they want and need, which can then lead to more effective interventions.
- Foster the emergence of therapeutic factors such as hope, and a corrective emotional experience.
- Make group process commentary which reflects to group members what they are saying and doing that is restricting them from making connections, or avoiding conflict instead of trying to resolve it, or other group resistances.
- Understand that the leader cannot be perceived as having favorites or showing favoritism as this can evoke transference such as sibling rivalry, narcissistic injury, and other harmful effects.
- Recognize the impact of the various cultural and diversity factors present in the group even when all members appear to be from the same culture, or diversity is not apparent.

There are other perceptual shifts that may be helpful as students begin to learn about group leadership.

Book Structure and Focus

Teaching practices are evolving and changing as more is learned about best and effective practices for teaching and learning. There is also the added complication of trying to teach concepts and practices that are complex, intangible, and that have nuances that are not easily defined or described. One example of what is meant can be seen for group therapy where there are conscious, nonconscious, and unconscious individual and group aspects in play at the same time and these must be taught and learned in the preparation of group leaders who have to be prepared to encounter a wide variety of group members together with their varied issues, problems and concerns. This is only one example of why instructors of group therapy may find it challenging to know what to present and how best to present the complexities and nuances that surround teaching and learning to be an effective group leader.

This book is written to help guide instructors to use substantiated effective teaching methods and techniques that incorporate didactic and experiential aspects that also take into account the learning styles of prospective group therapists and, in addition to understand the impact they can have on the group members. Among the teaching methods that are shown to be effective are active learning, concept mapping, flipping the classroom, just-in-time teaching, low-stakes testing, learning styles, mastery learning, peer instruction, team-based learning, and use of media. While not all of these will be appropriate for your course on group therapy, they are presented to give you some ideas that can make the teaching and learning more effective.

In presenting these, a metaphorical mixed media artwork model might be helpful as mixed media uses the concept of layers, various forms of symbols, and adapts to the wide variety of options available.

The first part of the book focuses on the premises for the teaching model, preparation for teaching group therapy that includes the teacher's prior learning and teaching experiences, planning and organizing the course, teaching techniques and strategies that the literature has shown to be effective. Most important are the descriptions for how the techniques may be used to facilitate learning for the students' inner leader self-development in addition to the knowledge base needed for effective group leadership, and proven group facilitation techniques and strategies. It is important to note that while there are group leaders in many settings such as meetings, team building and the like, and that facilitation can be similar in some respects, this book has a narrower focus on leadership for therapy groups that have 6–20 sessions and are not considered as long-term therapy groups. These therapy groups can be psychotherapy groups, psychoeducational groups, manualized groups, therapy groups, support or growth groups that are intended to guide group members in problem-solving, decisions making, more effective and satisfying interpersonal relationships, managing emotions and symptoms associated with psychiatric distress, emotional disturbances, medical conditions, and the like.

Suggested Course Organization

Planning is critical and essential and should be created to incorporate the components of the leadership/teaching model keeping in mind that the major thrust for teaching and learning is the development of the therapeutic self of the group leader. The other components are also important and the major thrust can be maintained when planning what and how to teach the group knowledge and techniques and skills components. Planning and organizing the course content includes ethical considerations, decisions about measurable goals and objectives, major learning components, teaching strategies and assessment.

Ethical Considerations

Do no harm is the prime ethical principle for teaching group therapy leadership. Ethical considerations guide the instructor in the selection of methods, techniques, and strategies. Just as in group therapy, the instructor has to attend to concerns such as confidentiality and privacy, freedom to exit, informed consent, dual roles and dual relationships, and to do no harm.

Since some or all of the same limits for *confidentiality and privacy* in therapy also apply to a course it is best if the instructor directly address these on the syllabus. There should be a clear statement on the syllabus that personal disclosures in class and in the T-group if used, are to be considered confidential and that students are prohibited from recording the class or T-group and posting any personal disclosures by classmates or the instructor on social media. The statement should also include the instructor's requirements for reporting such as the need to report violations of laws, licensure rule/laws, university policies and the like. Also note that anything requiring reporting to authorities will be discussed with the student before reporting. Acceptable postings can include the structure of the class, a description of activities, and their personal reactions and the like, but nothing about anyone else. Instructors should also have a clear statement about who will read assignments that include or that may include students' personal disclosures. It is best that graduate assistants do not read or grade assignments such as T-group journals or anything where students' disclosures are used.

One current ethical concern is about the use of mobile devices and their security. While the HIPAA standards provide for electronic protected health information, group leaders in training may not be as aware as needed of these standards, how information is stored and transmitted on their electronic devices that reduces the security and privacy of the information, the possibility of losing or having the device stolen or inadvertently viewed by others, the lack of security for publicly available Wi-Fi and cellular networks, and how to prevent unintentional sharing of confidential information.

A recommended practice which also has ethical implications that should be stated on the syllabus is that the students are in charge of their *self-disclosure* and are free to decide what and when to disclose. What is also recommended is that there be a clear statement that students will not be pushed to disclose personal sensitive material. Participation in a T-group should only require that students disclose their thoughts, feelings, and ideas about what is happening in the group in the here and now.

The syllabus and description of T-group can serve as documentation of *informed consent*. In other words, their continued enrollment in the class gives their consent to participate. As a part of informed consent on the syllabus can also state that students must discuss with the instructor if there are limits on their participation and to notify their therapists if they are in counseling.

Instructors should stay mindful of any *dual roles and dual relationships* they may have with students. An example of this is when the instructor leads a demonstration group where students may be concerned or have fears about their grades for either participating or not participating as the instructor is also their evaluator for the course. While the fears may be without merit, that does not lessen their impact on the person. It is also recommended that instructors be mindful of their roles as evaluators when leading demonstration groups as their experiences as group leaders may unintentionally lead them to deepen the emotional experiencing and disclosures of members in the demonstration groups. This is discussed in more detail in the section on demonstration groups in Chapter 2. Instructors are also advised to disclose other relationships they may have with a student or students in the class, such as a student who is also the instructor's graduate assistant and/or has been in a previous class or have other social connections.

Cultural and Diversity Concerns

Students and their future group members have both their own unique individual experiences and factors that affect their worldview and values. There is considerable diversity of beliefs, social structures, interactional patterns and expectations as well as the intersection of socioeconomic class, sexuality, gender identification and disability. Added to these are place of origin, educational level, racial/ethnic identity, marital status, citizenship status, age, employment and other important factors that comprise their self-identities. It can be helpful for students to become more aware of their implicit biases which in unconscious and unintentional but could play major roles for developing a therapeutic relationship, therapeutic ruptures, and unintentional microaggressions (van Nunspeet, Ellemers, & Derks, 2015).

This is one area where the instructor of the course can model the desired behaviors that shows respect for diversity and cultural differences. While differences should not be ignored or overlooked, neither should they be highlighted and featured. It can be best to let the student express or disclose their self-identify when they think that it is important to do so rather than the instructor pointing out these differences that are usually visible. Since groups tend to become cohesive around shared similarities and fail to do so around perceived differences, highlighting differences has implications for how the class or T-group becomes cohesive or fails to do so. The instructor's use of pronouns or indeterminate identifications can also be helpful to show prospective group leaders how to express concepts without using offensive identity language.

Syllabus Components

The major components for the syllabus are the goals and objectives, learning components, teaching strategies, and assessment. *Goals and objectives* are basic for deciding on other course components such as course content, sequencing, and activities. When developing the specific goals and objectives for the intended course, it can be helpful to keep three guiding questions in mind. What do you want group leaders in training to know refers to content material about groups such as stages of group development. What do you think is important for group leader to learn themselves and their roles in the group such as the critical components of the therapeutic self of the group leader that helps illustrate the complexity and value of leader understanding and knowledge for such things as knowing how to tune into the group as a whole, the interrelatedness of the layers of self to behaviors, attitudes, and actions in the group, and the importance of monitoring their countertransference? What and how to teach when and how to use group leadership skills to the benefit of the group and its members? Skills such as developing a therapeutic alliance, repairing therapeutic ruptures, fostering the emergence of group therapeutic factors and other group facilitation strategies.

It is helpful for the instructor to decide in advance what will be the *major learning components* for the class as these provide the basis for the assessment and evaluation of learning. Components for assessment and evaluation can include but are not limited to the following: tests, research papers, T-group observations and reflections, discussion groups, readings, review of webinars or other presentations, conference, and workshop attendance, and the like. These components should be specific and subject to objective evaluation processes and not rely solely on the instructor's judgment. It reduces some of the anxiety over course grades, allows students to better plan for the use of their time, and lessens some of the ambiguity and uncertainty.

There are numerous effective *teaching strategies* from which to choose. The next two chapters describe these in more detail but are listed here as possible choices. What is helpful is to select the teaching strategy best suited for the major goals and objectives. Proposed here is that strategies incorporate the developed inner therapeutic self where appropriate and try to focus on them intentionally in the particular teaching strategy chosen, and to try to embed something about this in every teaching technique when possible. Chapters 4–10 have examples for how to do this for particular topics for group therapy. Teaching strategies will include lectures, discussions, demonstration groups, T-group, case studies/situations, role play, journals and other writing to learn activities, creative activities, use of media, active learning, flipped the classroom, mastery learning, and other effective teaching strategies.

Planning also includes *assessment*. Assessment and evaluation can be both formal and informal. Formal assessment uses measures to evaluate the acquisition of knowledge. Examples of these measures are objective tests, essays, papers and other written documents. Most of these are traditional methods and are best used to assess surface learning and are useful for students' preparation for comprehensive, licensing, certifications and the like where the assessment strategy is a test. Informal assessment are methods that use other indicators of learning and growth, especially growth in application of knowledge and understanding. Some of the informal assessment strategies can be used as feedback to the student for improvement and are not necessarily a part of the formal grade for the course. Examples of some informal assessment indictors can be level of participation, and professionalism.

Current assessment strategies also utilize the widely accepted Bloom's Taxonomy as a guide for evaluation of surface and deeper learning. Bloom's (1956) initial taxonomy had the levels as knowledge, comprehension, application, analysis, synthesis, and evaluation. Subsequently, the level designations became remember, understand, apply, analyze, evaluate, and create where each higher level incorporates all of the previous levels. Using the latest designations remember is simple recall of learned materials, understand builds on recall to add an understanding of what was learned, apply expands on the first two levels to show how the learning can be used in new situations. Analyze assesses the ability to see and understand connections which brings in what was previously learned so as to be applicable in new and unknown situations. Evaluate incorporates appraisal, how to justify, selection, support, value, critique and defend, and the top level of create indicates that something new and novel is added. Assessment for learning group therapy will want to include all of the levels where possible and to use analysis and evaluate as much as possible.

Wiggins (1989) and others currently propose that there are other assessment strategies that can be better for assessment and evaluation of deep learning that extends beyond the first two levels in Bloom's Taxonomy of remembering and understanding. They propose alternative strategies that are termed authentic, constructivist/portfolio, and performance-based. Authentic assessment involves application of learning in a real-life scenario and is intended to reinforce both the surface learning of facts, and the deeper learning of understanding as they contribute to applications. Application is the third assessment level for Bloom's Taxonomy, as illustrated by the Constructivist/portfolio. Constructivist/portfolio has the student compile their work to demonstrate growth through their achievements which calls for reflection on how and why the achievements are evidence for growth and learning. Use of this method also allows for an exploration for future learning goals. Performance-based assessment uses analysis, evaluation, and creation, the top three levels of the taxonomy, to evaluate the extent to which knowledge, skills and strategy can be applied in context.

Tips for Organizing Instruction and Assessment

The following are some suggestions for possible course instructional strategies and assignments that can be used assessment based on the taxonomy:

- Lectures – tests using multiple-choice, true/false, fill in the blank, matching and essay can assess remembering and understanding of facts and other objective materials.

- Writing assignments for application – case studies, situations, discussions, observations.
- Writing assignments for analysis – readings, T-group journals, reviews.
- Embedded activities for personal growth and reflection and informal assessment such as professionalism– evaluation which is not a part of the grade.
- Performance based activities – leading a demonstration group, leading a discussion group, and observations for these can be for feedback only to suggest improvements.
- It is also important that the instructor identify the skills and abilities that students are expected to attain in the course and to relate these to the assessment strategies and how the elements that are assessed factor into the final grade. What is recommended to calm possible student fears about being negatively perceived and evaluated either by the instructor or classmates, is that some activities that call for input, disclosure, and the like not be a part of the formal assessment.

Overview of Chapters

The following is an overview of the major topics presented in the chapters.

In Chapter 1, "Teaching Group Therapy Components and Strategies", topics include the structure for the book, The 70–15–15 model, Group therapy knowledge factors, Group techniques and strategies, Layers of the teaching model, Course organization – ethical considerations, culture and diversity, goals and objectives, learning components, teaching strategies, assessment, Perceptual shifts.

In Chapter 2, "Current Evidence-based Teaching Practices", topics include current teaching practices, teaching strategies, group therapy focused teaching techniques and strategies – T-groups, journals (example), demonstration groups (guide, tip), role-play (tips and example), observing (tip), discussion groups (tip and examples), case study/situations (examples), reviews of readings, media, webinars (guidelines).

In Chapter 3, "Developing a Group Leader Therapeutic Self", major topics include the importance of the group leader's self, psychological boundaries, contributions to development of the inner self, and the importance of being self-reflective and for an emotional presence.

Chapter 4, "Organizing and Structuring the Group", includes topics on planning: Introduction, pre-group considerations, components for planning groups – children's groups, adolescents' groups, adults and older adults; assessment and evaluation, the critical first session –leader actions for the first session, sample outline for a first session, and the importance of planned group closure that includes premature termination.

Chapter 5, "Group Sessions and Members", describes group developmental stages, phases of member development, ethics and professional standards, culture and diversity in group therapy, culture and diversity awareness and competence, developing greater awareness and sensitivity, and strategies to increase the group pleader's cultural and diversity competence.

Chapter 6, "Therapeutic Components for Groups", presents group therapeutic factors and tips, fundamental relationship attributes, responding or communication competencies, group process and process illumination-indices of process, process topics – present centered focus, container, group dynamics, teaching members, constructive feedback, and judicious use; leadership tasks and skills, and process commentary skills.

Chapter 7, "Constructive Use of the Therapeutic Self", describes therapeutic attunement, developing a therapeutic alliance and Tips, Examples of therapeutic ruptures, why apologies do not work, suggestions for how to effectively atone for insensitivity and/or manage microaggressions, self-absorption in leader and members, and possible effects of leader self-absorption on group members.

Chapter 8, "Group Facilitation Process and Progress", examines empathic responding, identification of helpful but not empathic responses, empathic failures, group level empathic failures, cultural determinants and group culture, cultural social convention as a barrier, cultural social convention defenses, cultural social defenses and group communication patterns, cultural leader social defenses, and effects on group process commentary.

Chapter 9, "Managing Group Difficulties", describes narcissistic injury and its impact, conflict – a situation, a procedure, and group stages; member challenges – definitions and descriptions, leader contributions, examples of difficult member behaviors; constructive prevention strategies, counterproductive leader interventions, social psychology's deviant group member – importance and rationale, and deviant behavior and demeanor.

Chapter 10, "Intangible and Unseen Forces that Impact the Group", addresses group resistance and activities, scapegoating and tip, competition, seduction, tuning into group resistance, transference and counter-transference, metaphors, and promoting the corrective emotional experience.

Chapter 11, "Virtual and Restricted-Setting Therapy Groups", describes benefits and challenges, planning and organizing sessions, technology requirements, options for sessions, the leader's space, ethics and professional issues,–confidentiality and privacy, documentation and required reporting, state and federal laws, and scope of practice; managing group dynamics, group level dynamics, use of activities, and the importance of an orientation session.

Chapter 12, "Emerging Group Therapy Concerns and Possibilities", examines cybersecurity actions to protect group leaders and members, AI for instruction, AI for group therapy: definitions and descriptions, background for therapeutic use, advantages – personalized care, shorter wait times, removes barriers, boosts efficiency, monitoring, accuracy of diagnosis and treatment, reduced costs, augments the capabilities of differently abled individuals, AI modalities – conversational AI, embodied AI, 24/7, speech enabled applications, speech based applications, personalizing, ethics and other issues – privacy, surveillance, autonomy, bias and discrimination.

References

AGPA & IBCGP. (2002). *Guidelines for Ethics in Group Psychotherapy*. New York: American Group Psychotherapy Association & International Board of Certified Group Psychotherapists.

Bloom, B.S. (1956) *Taxonomy of Educational Objectives Handbook: The Cognitive Domain*. New York: David McKay.

Brown, N. (1992) *Teaching Group Dynamics*. Greenport, CT: Praeger.

van Nunspeet, F., Ellemers, N., & Derks, B. (2015). Reducing implicit bias: How moral motivation helps people refrain from making "automatic" prejudiced associations. *Translational Issues in Psychological Science*, 1(4), 382–391. doi:10.1037/tps0000044.

Wiggins, G, (1989) A true test: Toward more authentic and equitable assessment. *The Phi Delta Kappan*, 70(9), 703–713.

Yalom, I. & Leszcz, M. (2021). *The Theory and Practice of Group Psychotherapy* (6th edition). New York: Basic Books.

2 Current Evidence–Based Teaching Practices

Current Teaching Practices

Evidence-based teaching practices (Petty, 2006) or best teaching practices (McLaughlin & Mandin, 2001) fall into six categories. Instructors for the group course may find some of these to be valuable to enhance learning:

1 Cooperative learning – working in small groups during class on a task or activities.
2 Assessment for learning – provide feedback to modify teaching and learning activities, and to improve teaching.
3 Reciprocal teaching – using students as teachers in small groups.
4 Whole class interactive – knowledge is created by all students in a class together in an interactive and collaborative way mediated by the instructor.
5 Concept driven teaching – an iterative process of constantly pulling apart ideas, putting them back together, reapplying to different situations, correcting misconceptions, and using information to estimate, reason, evaluate and judge.
6 Visual presentations and graphic organizers – use of both text and visuals to show relationships and connections between concepts, terms, and facts, and promotes creative thinking.

These practices rely heavily on student participation, having the instructor organize each class session in advance to involve the students in learning the cognitive material, student interactions either in dyads or small groups, targeted and consistent assessment and feedback, less reliance on tests, and use of relevant real-world applications. All of these evidence-based teaching practices are incorporated into the next two sections on teaching strategies, and group focused teaching techniques and strategies.

Teaching Strategies

The following strategies that are described also have examples for how these can be used to teach group therapy concepts and practices, guide students in safe self-exploration, and deepen their understanding of some of

DOI: 10.4324/9781003329787-2

the intangibles associated with group therapy and group leadership. The ten teaching strategies described are derived from current and former studies that support their efficacy. The strategies described are active learning, flipped the classroom, concept mapping, just-in-time teaching, low stakes testing, mastery learning, peer instruction, team-based learning, use of media, writing to learn.

Active learning is the instructional strategy that involves the student to take an active role in the classroom. The instructor provides instructional activities that require students to do things and to think about what they are doing. Freeman et al. (2014) describe it as focusing on higher order thinking to participate in activities such as discussions, making class presentations, and other interactions with classmates. They are asked to think about their personal learning. Among the examples provided are the following.

- Pause during lectures and ask students to discuss and revise their notes in pairs.
- Retrieval practice also uses a pause in the lecture to ask students to write everything they remember from the previous 15–18-minute class segment.
- Demonstrations of procedures, processes, concepts, and the like.
- Think–pair–share is the strategy where the instructor ask students to pose a higher-order question to then share with a classmate for two minutes which is followed with an explanation by the instructor.
- Peer instruction occurs when students are given a question to answer, then formed into groups for a discussion to produce a group response, the responses from the groups are posted, and the instructor provides additional explanation or information.
- Minute papers start with the instructor asking a question that calls for reflection or critical thinking. The process is then to share responses, discuss, and collect.
- Strip sequence is a strategy to determine if students know the steps for a procedure or process.
- Steps are written on strips and students have to put them in the correct order.
- Concept maps are visual representations of relationships between concepts placed in nodes which are usually circles, labeled arrows show connections between key concepts.
- Mini maps are lists of concepts to incorporate into a concept map where there are numerous concepts that could apply.
- Categorizing grids can be used when there are several important categories and lists of terms, images, and the like that students then put into the correct categories.
- Decision making where students have to justify a decision.
- Case based learning incorporates students deciding what is relevant for the case, other needed information, and what will be the impact of their decision.

Flipped classroom is a strategy that can be described as inverted learning (Toriz, 2019). Online platforms are used as part of the class, learning is delivered through video and other media such as readings, and class time is used for collaborative learning. Thus, most of the instruction is not based on teaching delivered lectures but occurs out of class and is the responsibility of the student.

Concept mapping uses visual diagrams to illustrate relationships between items such as techniques, cognitive categories and the like. These are usually presented in circles with arrows used to show the connections.

Just-in-time teaching also uses the internet and computers for teaching, and where a considerable amount of the instruction occurs out of class. The intent is to encourage student reading assignments and complete other work out of class and the instructor uses class time to focus on posing questions for discussion about the assigned material, or can give quizzes at the beginning of class, and students are asked to integrate and analyze information from other classes. (Li, Ling, & Tan, 2021)

Low stakes testing uses continual assessment for feedback on learning (Gray, 2020). Questions, and problems and the like are embedded in videos and lectures and the students have to submit their responses which are graded and/or feedback given. The rationales for frequent quizzes and the like are that this promotes involvement with the material to be learned, prepares students for tests, and the instructor can better understand gaps in learning and correct misunderstandings.

Mastery learning is also known as competency based (Bisggard et al., 2018). This method requires that competency be clearly defined, is evidence based, and that there be observable behavioral changes. The steps toward competence have to be sequential and include deliberate practice with feedback. The competencies are specific and rigid, such as requiring a sequence of steps for mastery.

Peer instruction is a form of cooperative learning (Crouch & Mazur, 2001). The instructor prepares materials to be read before class that require written responses that are either submitted prior to class or after class. These materials may include questions, case studies, situations, readings and the like. The material such as questions are then discussed in class in groups that are peer led where the peer explains answers to their classmates. Another version is where students make a short in–class presentation, questions about the presentation are asked with students given 2 minutes for a written response. The answers are then presented to a nearby classmate and discussed.

Team-based methods require that the class be formed into teams that will work together for the duration of the class (Brown, 2000; Michelsen & Sweet, 2011). The teams work on application activities that are designed to promote critical thinking and team development. Peer evaluation is also a part of this method.

Use of social media is evolving as a teaching method (Bexheti et al., 2014). Social media has four teaching advantages – students are able to access a large amount of materials, they can create digital content, the connections to share knowledge, and collaboration can be fostered. Other advantages are that the various social media platforms are familiar to students and provides opportunities to create and share. Among the disadvantages are the ethical concerns for privacy and confidentiality, ownership of intellectual property, lack of instructor monitoring and other safety measures, and the possibility of trolling and other such actions. There may also be legal concerns.

Writing to learn as a teaching method has considerable evidence for its efficacy to promote learning (Chmarkh, 2020). It is described as short informal writing about key concepts and ideas. The Langer and Applebee (1987) study determined that the method produces more learning, it can focus on different kinds of information, and promotes more complex and thoughtful inquiry. MacDonald and Cooper (1992) found writing helpful for academic journals, and Cannon (1990) found it useful to incorporate personal journals into the course.

Both the teaching practices and strategies described are intended to encourage critical thinking, higher order thinking and inquiry, promote student involvement and interactions, and to reduce complexity. They emphasize that the learner is an important component for teaching and have produced numerous ways to accomplish these goals. The next section describes group focused teaching techniques and strategies that can be specifically applied to teaching group therapy.

Group Therapy Focused Teaching Techniques and Strategies

Group focused teaching techniques presented in this section are lectures, T-groups, journals, demonstration groups, role-play, observing, discussion, case studies/situations, and reviews as these are applied to group therapy. Examples are provided for teaching and relating to group therapy, and guides for implementing.

Lectures

There are advantages to using lectures for teaching and learning. Lectures usually occur when the instructor or designated person delivers information to students which is a unidirectional dissemination of information (Bligh, 2000). Among the advantages of lectures ae that they deliver a large amount of information, the presenter can collect and collate information from a variety of sources, and it is a method to explain complexities and share expert opinions (Matheson, 2008). Among the disadvantages are that lectures are not useful to effect changes for attitudes and behaviors, or to learn how to think consistent with the discipline, and results in passive learning which has been found to not be as effective as is active learning (Bligh, 2000).

Miller et al. (2013) found that lectures are more beneficial for learning when they also include some hands-on interactive activities such as discussions and creative activities that call for all students to participate. Eze and Edward (2017) found that attention spans for lectures are 15–20 minutes and recommend that lectures be limited to that frame.

Tip: Teaching tips for group therapy applications for lectures would include keeping the lectures brief, provide information about a limited number of topics for each class session, and examples for how the information may be used and applied. Some topics that will lend themselves to lectures include a history of group therapy and psychotherapy, ethical concerns, a rationale for the importance of cultural and diversity group concepts, stages of group development, definitions for group therapeutic factors, steps for conflict resolution, and may other group related topics. Keeping the lectures brief allows for time to include other learning experiences to reinforce and expand the concepts from the lecture, and to involve the personal associations of students. Other learning experiences such as discussions, demonstrations, activities, and role play can be useful adjuncts for lectures.

T-Groups

A T-group or Training group is a form of group training where group members learn about leadership, group dynamics, and group membership skills in a small group that emphasizes here and now experiencing and reactions, and the giving and receiving of feedback by group members. T-groups were founded by Kurt Lewin (1944) as a part of the National Training Laboratories created by the Office of Naval Research and the National Education Association in 1947. This form of training was developed according to Lewin's model of experiential learning.

T-groups have several commonalties with therapy groups including but not limited to the importance of the therapeutic alliance, membership may be voluntary or involuntary, the main focus is on the here and now, although their past experiences may be associated with present experiencing, members' personal goals and objectives can be a focus, therapeutic group factors ae encouraged to emerge, and the group may experience the group therapy development stages.

Major differences with therapy groups include the role of the group leader, group members are in charge of their disclosures and are not pushed to disclose, although the past may be tapped, it is the present here and now experiencing that is the emphasis and focus, there is no formal screening for placement in the group, members do not receive diagnoses or assessment, no treatment plans or planning is developed, there are no predetermined topics for group sessions as the group determines the topic for the session, interactions are encouraged among group members, and there is less reliance on the leader to direct the session.

Members of T-groups are considered to be observers and participants. Learning occurs from observation of self and others, exploring personal reactions that emerge in the session(s), and from giving and receiving constructive feedback. Group sessions can be a rich source for learning about oneself. In addition, the sessions provide opportunities to learn about group process and procedures. Among the many aspects of group that will emerge in sessions are the importance of identifying empathic failures and effecting their repair, learning how to tune into group process such as identifying the session's theme, and/or group level resistance, the metaphors that may emerge, and other important invisible forces that can affect the group and its members. Other learning opportunities include learning how to how to make group process comments, the importance of monitoring and managing countertransference, the impact and importance of culture and diversity issues and concerns and how these can affect members and the group, assistance to build a therapeutic self through understanding relationships and communications among group members and with the leader.

There are many variations for T-groups. The previous description used the T-groups for an academic purpose that incorporates some personal learning and there are other ways to organize the experience. For example, the experience could be over a long and intensive weekend where the group sessions are interspersed with some didactics, but the primary focus is on personal learning. Another variation is to only have the group meet for part of a semester or quarter. Students could also be instructed to attend groups in other settings such as at a counseling center at a university. The goals and purpose for the T-group as well as other course demands will determine the best structure for the duration for the group.

T-groups when used as described for a class over a semester or quarter where students attend for 8–12 weekly sessions can also be used for academic learning of group intangibles and some group facilitation skills and, when combined with journals as described in the next section, can be a valuable assessment tool.

Journals

Much of the recent literature on using journals as a part of classroom teaching gathered data and other information from the journals students wrote for their personal growth group experiences and were focused on self-reflection (Woodbridge & O'Beirne, 2017; Ziomek-Daigle, 2017).

Commonalities among the studies were the use of journals and the use of qualitative research design and analysis. Only one study was found that used a quasi-experimental design (Ohrt, Robinson, & Hagedorn, 2012). Most researchers noted that the journals were used for self-reflection.

Luke and Kiweewa (2010) conducted a qualitative study where weekly reflective journals were analyzed and found that students identified 30 aspects of the group that they felt contributed to their personal growth. Ohrt et al. (2014) followed 52 group members' development through 10 weekly journals, Steen et al. (2014) used web-based journals to explore changes in cohesion within experiential growth groups and found that group cohesion decreased from pretest to posttest, and Young et al. (2013) surveyed 43 personal growth group participants and concluded that there was evidence that participants do learn about essential group processes.

Ohrt, Robinson, and Hagedorn (2012) conducted a quasi-experimental study to compare the valuing of group therapeutic factors between participants in personal growth groups and participants in psychoeducational groups. Both groups have similar valuing of these factors.

There is little or no research on effective methods for teaching how to identify and capitalize on group dynamics. This is an important consideration for preparing group leaders to work in the variety of settings, and with varying target audiences who will have differing characteristics and conditions that they will encounter. While group dynamics can be described in isolation, the challenge for group leaders in training is to be able to identify these as they appear in real time in the group as a whole. The challenges are many – dynamics do not appear in isolation they are ever shifting and changing in the session, they can be exhibited differently for the different group members, and the leader has to attend to all of this at the same time, plus leaders need to understand these so as to provide effective interventions (Brown, 2011). One means for teaching the dynamics of the group as a whole for mental health professionals is through the use of a training group (T-group) experience as part of the learning process (Gans et al., 2002; Scheidlinger, 2004).

Example and tip: Following is an example of how T-group experiences were reported vial a journal that focused on academics that can be ethically assessed and evaluated. Students were required to report on their observations of the following T-group factors and experiencing. Each factor also has a description.

1   List and describe effective group member behaviors. Sample effective behaviors included having a focus for the session and openness to giving and receiving feedback.
2   List and describe counterproductive member behaviors. Sample ineffective behaviors included waiting to become involved in the group, not participating, and chronic tardiness.
3   List personal feelings experienced throughout the session (Brown, 2011). No explanation or exploration of feelings were required.
4   List personal resistances (Rutan et al., 2014). Resistances were identified as refusal to contribute to a discussion because it was too sensitive or distressing, or not responding. Again, no explanation or exploration was required.
5   Feelings directly expressed by group members. The direct expression had to be naming or labeling of a feeling, and not an inference of the feeling(s).
6   Empathic failures. These can be external, such as a member not receiving a reflective or empathic response or there is a change of topic

after providing the member made an emotional disclosure or expressed an intense feeling. These may also be internal such as becoming bored or thinking that a disclosure is surface or trivial (Brown, 2021; Kohut, 1977).

7   Empathic failure repair (Brown, 2021; Kohut, 1977). These were defined as noting that someone did not receive a reflective or empathic response and providing a belated response that acknowledges the feeling that did not receive the reflective or empathic response. An apology was not a repair.

This is one way to incorporate learning through writing about groups into academic projects that can be objectively assessed and evaluated. Journal writing can also be used for self-reflection such as critiques for student's leadership when they facilitate a group, as a means to better identify possible countertransference, and as a means for their deeper self-exploration but which is not graded.

Demonstration Groups

The demonstration group is a teaching technique that allows for immersion in the experience for learning concepts and processes that involves both observation and participation (Gans et al., 2002). Generally, demonstration groups in classes are formed of a number of volunteers from the class while the remaining students observe. The basic components for a demonstration group are a clearly defined goal and purpose, the volunteer group participants, the group leader who can be a student or the instructor, directions and orientation for the experience, the outside of the group observers, and the debriefing.

The goal and purpose for the demonstration should be clearly defined and described prior to implementation. What concepts and/or process is the focus and emphasis for the demonstration should be explained. For example, a demonstration group could be formed for the goal and purpose of having students experience what occurs when there are difficult group member behaviors such as storytelling. While students can imagine what it would be like to participate or try to lead during the storytelling, experiencing it in a demo group can provide an expanded and deeper understanding of the impact of that behavior on the leader, the group members, and the group as a whole.

Guide for implementation: One of the first tasks for the instructor is to decide who will lead the group. Many instructors may want to demonstrate their understanding and expertise and will be the leader for the demonstration group. This stance can produce the difficulty of dual roles where the instructor is both the evaluator and as the group leader is in the position of asking students to disclose what may be sensitive and hurtful personal material. Students can be apprehensive about pleasing the instructor and how participating in the group will affect their grade for the course which puts them in an awkward position. The other two possibilities are to have a student lead the group for practice, or to have a leaderless demo group. Either of these can work for the main purpose for the demonstration of the particular concept or process. This can also provide the instructor with the opportunity to highlight the important actions related to the purpose and goal.

It is best to ask for volunteers rather than assigning students to participate. The instructor can first state the goal and purpose and then ask for a certain number of volunteers. The number of members of the demo group can be dependent on the time available for the class as there has to be adequate time to brief the participants, the observers, institute the demonstration, and then debriefing and summary. While it may take time for the demo group to jell so that the concept can be demonstrated, there also needs to be adequate time for the debriefing and summary.

The instructor should provide instructions and orientation for both the participants and the observers. Among the instructions are the time that is allotted for the demonstration, what is expected of the participants, what the demon group leader will do as part of the demonstration, the participants' freedom to choose what and how much to disclose. A general guideline for their participation is to ask that participants express their thoughts, feelings, and ideas in the here and now group experiencing. Basic instructions for the observers are to note and be ready to describe their reactions and thoughts, identifiers of the purpose for the demonstration, and other group as a whole factors, but not to focus on any one demo group member or to make evaluative comments. Evaluative comments include should, ought, good, bad, right, or wrong. Ask them to just report what they observed and what they personally experienced.

It is essential that there be sufficient time for debriefing the participants. It may also be a good practice to debrief the participants before opening the discussion up to the observers. Debriefing participants can also provide some information that is related to the concept. Asking what it was like to be in the group, to being observed, and how they may have experienced the concept that was the focus of the demonstration helps them to transition out of the experience and back to the classroom. Debriefing the observers can ask them what they observed, their reactions during the portrayal, what was triggered or evoked for them as they watched, and other such explorations that will personalize the observation for them. Block any questions posed by observers to participants.

Tip: Techniques such as empathic responding, identifying empathic failures and their repair, a corrective emotional experience, promoting some group therapeutic factors such as universality, and recognizing existential factors in a session can be use for demonstrations. There are numerous other such group concepts, techniques and strategies that can form the basis for a demonstration.

Role play

Role play can be used in a wide variety of contexts and content areas (Rao & Stupans, 2012). Sogunro (2004) describes it as taking on specific roles and act out a case-based scenario to learn content, ambiguous and complex concepts, or to deepen their understanding. Bobbit et al. (2001) and Rosa (2012) consider role play to be better for college students that are traditional methods. There is considerable research on its effectiveness and best practices (Maier, 2002; Rao & Stupans, 2012) report that it is effective in the three learning domains of affective, cognitive, and behavioral. Westrup and Planander (2013) found that role playing contributes to better understanding of others' perspective, become more empathic and can lead to greater self-reflection and awareness as well as practicing a skill. McEwen et al. (2014) propose that role play leads to a deeper understanding of the cognitive material. Finally, using role-play can promote change behaviors and use best practices in real-world settings (Beard et al., 1995).

Pavey and Donoghue (2003, p. 7) summarize the benefits of using role-play "to get students to apply their knowledge to a given problem, to reflect on issues and the views of others, to illustrate the relevance of theoretical ideas by placing them in a real-world context, and to illustrate the complexity of decision-making". Role play as a teaching technique has been used in various fields such as medicine, law, business and psychology (Westrup & Planander, 2013). In educational settings it is generally used with an emphasis on the social dynamic of learning and fostering collaboration among students (Joyce & Weil, 2000), helps students to better grasp practical cognitive skills (Shapiro & Leopold, 2012), and (Westrup & Planander, 2013) found that it increases student engagement and knowledge retention.

Rao and Stupans (2012) created three ways to use role play as a teaching technique: Role-Switch, Acting, and Almost Real Life. Role-Switch requires the student to assume the role of another person to better understand that person's actions and motivations, of someone else. Acting provides for an opportunity to practice newly developed skills by using a situation where the skill could be applicable. Almost Real Life is a role-play that used as much of a real experience as possible while keeping the role players safe. Rao and Stupans also recommend that instructors using role play as a teaching technique first reflect on the learning goals of the role-play and choosing a case that best reaches those goals; ensure that both the instructor and students are adequately prepared with case materials and familiar with what the concept or skills intended to be learned are, and have sufficient time available for feedback and debriefing. Disadvantages of using role play include the amount of time available for first orienting the students to what is being acted out, the actions for the role play, and debriefing.

Tips and examples: Role play can be a valuable teaching technique. Among the situations that can be portrayed are dreams where the dreamer portrays each item in the dream including inanimate objects, as behavioral rehearsal for an upcoming dreaded event, and as a conflict. One alternative way to set up a role play is to have the person who has the dilemma or problem be the director of the action but not to participate in it. The director selects the people to play the different roles, prepares them for the role by describing their contributions, characteristics, and actions and then allows them to reenact the event or problem. After the role play is completed, the director is asked how accurate the portrayal was— usually it is very accurate even with the minimal orientation – and then each member in the portrayal is debriefed with an emphasis on what was triggered for them, and finally, the observers are debriefed. Using this method, not only does the director learn something about their problem, issue, or concern, but the players and observers also gain some personal insights.

It can also be insightful when used to better understand a dream where the person with the dream acts out each element in the dream and then makes associations. Observers of this kind of role play can also contribute to understanding by reporting on what was evoked for them as they watched.

Observing

Observing is usually a passive role but can be enhanced when specific directions are provided for what is to be observed (Weiss & Rutan, 2016). This can make it more relevant for learning course material especially the intangibles found in group therapy. The instructor can provide a framework for the observations, as well as the time for each observer to report. The following components are recommended for observations.

- *External* – Describe what behaviors are to be observed and reported on for individuals and for the group as a whole. It is important to try to always have students observe the entire group and not just single out individuals.
- *Internal* – Part of the observations should be what thoughts, feelings, and other reactions were evoked during the observations. By observing both externally and internally students can learn to automatically check-in with their own experiencing and learn how to use this to better understand what is happening in the group.
- *Nonverbal communications* – A significant part of what can be observed are the nonverbal communications for individuals, among group members, and with the group leader. It can be helpful to direct the observers to report on behavior that was observed and to not make judgments or inferences about that behavior.
- *Resistance* – It can also be important that observers attend to their personal resistance that is triggered as well as observing indicators of resistance in the group. It may be best to not have observers report on how individuals demonstrated resistance but to have them report on indices of resistance by the group as a whole. For example, resistance such as abruptly

changing the topic and the group goes along with the change could be observed as there was an abrupt change of topic but not label it as resistance or identify the person who made the topic change.

- *Verbal expressions* – Observing verbal expressions of thoughts and feelings produces some objectivity and can help students learn to not make inferences, derive implications, or speculate on possible reasons for what was said. It can be very helpful for students to learn to focus on observable and verifiable behaviors rather than intangibles such as attitudes.

- *Effective and counterproductive behaviors* – Observing behaviors that were helpful to the group's progress can be seen as effective and the behaviors that are counterproductive can be clues for what needs to be addressed in the group. Again, try to not have the focus be on individual group members and labelling them, try to focus on general behaviors by group members. Examples of effective group behaviors are interacting with individual group members such as speaking directly to the person, a willingness to verbalize current feelings and thoughts, and taking responsibility for personal feelings. Examples of counterproductive behaviors are waiting to become involved in the session, becoming distracted, and directing communications through the leader instead of directly to group members.

Tip: Instructors must be very careful in how they instruct observers to give feedback. The tendency is for students to give compliments and to ignore actions that could be counterproductive and show a need for improvement. Further, some students being observed may be hypervigilant and overly sensitive to any hint of perceived criticisms. It can be a tricky balance to illustrate for them how the feedback can be effectively used for improvement and to also take care of their feelings about not being perfect.

Discussion Groups

Discussion groups in the classroom have some advantages and disadvantages (Kivlighan & Chatman, 2018). Among the advantages are that the discussion allows the instructor to identify misunderstandings, highlight where students' lack experience and information, can show the depth and breadth of understanding gained, extent of personal associations, suggest new avenue to explore, and provide an opportunity for them to practice leadership. Disadvantages are that all students may not participate in the discussion or say things like, "I don't have anything to add", the amount of time available for a full discussion and follow-up, may not add to the body of knowledge about the topic, the discussion may not stay on track or topic, and irrelevances can be introduced during the discussion.

The discussions will be more useful if the following are used for preparation, initiation, and follow-up for discussions: identify a focus for the discussion, prepare the designated leader, identify expected discussion group members' participation, ask discussants to provide examples, prepare a list of questions/topics as a guide, debrief, and summarize. Discussions are more fruitful when they are focused on an identifiable group therapy/facilitation topic. It is important that the focus remain on topics relevant to the goals and purpose for the class. Instructors may want to lead the discussion and that can be helpful to encourage participation as well as maintaining the focus for the discussion. An alternative to having the instructor as the discussion group leader is to designate a student to be the leader and give them sufficient instructions on how to facilitate the discussion.

Discussion groups can be listed as a class expectation in the syllabus which gives the instructor an opportunity to describe the expectations for participation such as to volunteer their input, to give examples related to their group experiences or other experiences, to directly respond to other group members, and to reflect other members' feelings. Preparation for a student group leader would include a clear statement that they are not expected to teach the topic, to start and end the discussion on time, provide a framework for the discussion such as to begin the discussion with stating the purpose, the time available for the discussion and how members can voice their input, e.g. use the reaction button on the screen if the discussion is virtual, raise hands, etc.

Tip: Following are some examples to give the group leaders ideas about what to ask as prompts for the discussion. It can be important that the student leader have time to think about what to ask and how to present it.

- *"I found _____ to be the most interesting point for me. What was most interesting for you?"*
- *Another prompt would be to note what information was new, different, or surprising for you and then ask group members to respond.*
- *"What information do you think will be most useful for you as a group leader."*
- *"What was not clear or needs more information."*

An example: Depending on the number of students in the class it could also be helpful to designate the students who are not in the discussion group as observers. They would be given instructions similar to the following and provided an opportunity to provide feedback on their observations and the prompts.

1   *Write your answers to the prompts and be prepared to present these after the discussion group ends.*
2   *Note what feelings were directly expressed by the discussants.*
3   *Be prepared to volunteer your input. If you do not volunteer, the instructor will call on you as all observers are expected to respond.*

The instructor can also summarize the thoughts, feelings and ideas that were expressed by group members and the observers and provide some direct connections to the topic.

Case Studies/Situations

A learning technique is to have students apply some group concepts to group situations that are commonly encountered. The following three examples use writing for responses. The directions for the responses for the examples are below.

Directions: Provide an intervention for the described group situation.

1 Assume that you are the group leader.
2 The members of the group are similar to those in your T-group.
3 Your proposed intervention must be implemented in the group session. No taking a member aside or meeting with them outside of the group.
4 The intervention you propose must be consistent with text(s) materials.
5 Assume the situation arises in the 4th or 5th session after the group is under way.
6 Provide a minimum of a one-page answer for the proposed intervention.
7 Describe a group level process and procedure for the conflict.

Directions should also be provided for what is supposed to be in their answers.

Example 1

Sally and Eleanor are openly disagreeing on an issue currently in the news. Neither one seems to be listening to the other person. The conflict has been going on for some time in the session. Other group members say little, but some appear to be taking sides by their non-verbal behaviors. The group is tense, and members seem uncomfortable. As the leader, what would you do or say?

Example 2

The group does not seem to be able to settle on a topic in this 5th session. The discussion keeps ranging on many out of the group topics and issues. Members seem to be content to just chit chat. How would you intervene as the group leader?

Although verbally responding in class can be used, there are two advantages for having students write the response. By using writing for the responses, the answers are usually unique to the student responding and are not confounded by hearing what others say which give the instructor a better idea of the student's knowledge and understanding. In addition, the written responses can be used as assessment.

Reviews (Readings, Media, Webinars)

It is impossible for any textbook to provide all of the information available relative to group therapy as new information emerges constantly, there are page and word limits on what can be presented in a book, and there are other nuances that other resources can provide such as readings, media, and webinars. Instructors can incorporate new and emerging materials, reviews of some historical information and findings and expand the understanding of concepts with a variety of perspectives. Written reviews of readings, media, webinars and even some conferences can help clarify what the student learned and understood, their personal associations and connections to the material, provide a means for assessing learning, help identify misunderstandings and lack of information, and are means for expanding learning by using current information. The instructor should provide a framework for the review that emphasizes the content and how this applies or is related to group therapy and/or group leadership.

Example and tip: Following is an example of directions for reporting on readings. There are four sections to the review: theme, intervention, knowledge, and expertise.

1   *Theme – Provide the theme of the article in one brief sentence, phrase, or word.*
2   *Intervention – Describe how the group leader can use the information from the article to decide on an intervention.*
3   *Discuss briefly the most important piece of knowledge you gained from the article – knowledge.*
4   *Describe your experiences or encounter with the subject or theme of the reading including one or more feelings then, and one or more feelings now as you recall and write your answer.*

Technical aspects:

a   *Use the four headings theme, intervention, knowledge gained and your experiences, and present your answers for each separately.*
b   *There must be a minimum of two full pages in APA format. No maximum number of pages.*
c   *Resources other than another person may be consulted.*

Additional sections for a review could include asking for examples, other applications, how the group characteristics and needs could be important to identify, and even for personal associations.

References

Beard, R.L., Salas, E., & Prince, C. (1995). Enhancing transfer of training: Using role-play to foster teamwork in the cockpit. *The International Journal of Aviation Psychology*, 5(2), 131–143.

Bexheti, L., Ismali, & B. Cico (2014). *An analysis of social media usage in teaching and learning.* Presented at the International Conference on Circuits, Systems, Signal Processing, Communications and Computers.

Bligh, D. A. (2000). *What's the Use of Lectures?* San Francisco, CA: Jossey-Bass.

Bisggard, C. S.Rubak, S.Rodt, J.Petersen, & P. Musaeus (2018). The effects of graduate competency-based education and mastery learning on patient care and return on investment: a narrative review of basic anesthetic procedures. *BMC Medical Education*, 13(154). doi:10.1186/s12909-12018-1262-1267.

Bobbit, L.M., Inks, S.A., Kemp, K.J. & Mayo, D.T. (2001). Integrating marketing courses to enhance team-based experiential learning. *Journal of Marketing Education*, 22 (1), 15–24.

Brown, N. (2000) *Creating High Performance Classroom Groups*. New York: Taylor & Francis.

Brown, N. W. (2009). *Becoming a Group Leader*. Upper Saddle River, NJ: Pearson Education.

Brown, N. (2011). *Psychoeducational Groups* (3rd edition). New York: Routledge.

Brown, N. (2021). The significance and importance of repairing empathic failures. In Y. I. Kane, S. Masselink, & A. Weiss (Eds.), *Women, Intersectionality and Power in Group Psychotherapy*. New York: Routledge.

Cannon, R. (1990). Experiments with writing to teach microbiology. *The American Biology Teacher*, 52(3), 156–158. doi:10.2307/4449068.

Chmarkh, M (2020). "Writing to learn" research: A synthesis of empirical studies. *European Journal of Educational Research* 85–96. doi:10.12873/en-jer.10.1.85/10(1).

Crouch, C. & E. Mazur (2001). Peer instruction: Ten years of experience and results. *American Journal of Physics*. 69(9), 970–977. doi:10.119/1.1374249.

Eze, C. & O. Edwards (2017). Lecture duration: A risk factor for quality teaching and learning in higher education. *Integrity Journal of Education and Training* 1(1), 1–5.

Freeman, S., *et al.* (2014). Active learning increases student performance in science, engineering, and mathematics. *PNAS*, 111(23), 8410–8415. doi:10.1073/pnas.1319030111.

Gans, J. S., Rutan, J. S., & Lape, E. (2002). The demonstration group: A tool for observing group process and leadership style. *International Journal of Group Psychotherapy*, 52(2), 233–252. doi:10.1521/ijgp.52.2.233.45502.

Gray, S. (2020). Embedded video questions as a low stake assignment during remote learning transition. *Journal of Chemical Education*, 97(9), 3172–3175. doi:10.1021/ACS.jchemed0c00505.

Joyce, B. R., & Weil, M. (2000). Role playing; studying social behavior and values. In B. R. Joyce, M. Weil, & E. Calhoun (Eds.), *Models of Teaching* (6th ed., pp. 57–75). Boston, MA: Allyn and Bacon.

Kivlighan, D. M., & Chapman, N. A. (2018). Extending the multicultural orientation (MCO) framework to group psychotherapy: A clinical illustration. *Psychotherapy*, 55(1), 39–44. doi:10.1037/pst0000142.

Kohut, H. (1977). *The Restoration of the Self.* Madison, CT: International Universities Press.

Lewin, K. (1944). Dynamics of group action. *Educational Leadership*, 1, 195–200.

Langer, J., & Applebee, A. (1987). *How Writing Shapes Thinking: A Study of Teaching and Learning*. Urbana, IL: National Council of Teachers of English.

Li, J., Ling, & Tan, L. C. (2021). *Blending peer instruction with just-in-time teaching: Jointly optimal task scheduling with feedback for classroom flipping*. Presented at the Eighth ACM Conference on Learning.

Luke, M., & Kiweewa, J. (2010). Personal growth and awareness of counseling trainees in an experiential group. *Journal for Specialists in Group Work*, 35(4), 365–388. doi:10.1080/01933922.2010.514976.

MacDonald, S. P., & Cooper, C. R. (1992). Contribution of academic and dialogic journals to writing about literature. In A. Herrington & C. Moran (Eds.), *Writing, Teaching, and Learning in the Disciplines* (pp. 137–155). New York: Modern Language Association.

Maier, H.W. (2002). Role playing: structures and educational objectives. Retrieved from www.cyc-net.org/cyc-online/cycol-0102-roleplay.html.

Matheson, C. (2008). The educational value and effectiveness of lectures. *The Clinical Teacher*, 5, 218–221.

McEwen, L., A. Stokes, K. Crowley & C. Roberts (2014) Using role-play for expert science communication with professional stakeholders in flood risk management. *Journal of Geography in Higher Education*, 38(2), 277–300. doi:10.1080/03098265.2014.911827.

McLaughlin, K. & H. Mandin (2001). A schematic approach to diagnosing and resolving lecturalgia. *ASME Medical Education*, 35(12), 1135–1142. doi:10.1046/j.1365-2923.2002.01090.x.

Michelsen, L. & Sweet, M. (2011). Team based learning. *New Directions for Teaching and Learning*, 128, 41–51. doi:10.1002/1.467.

Miller, C. J., McNear, J., Metz, M. J. (2013). A comparison of traditional and engaging lecture methods in a large, professional-level course. *Advances in Physiology Education*, 37, 347–355.

Ohrt, J. H., Robinson, E. H., & Hagedorn, W. B. (2012). Group leader development: Effects of personal growth and psychoeducational groups. *Journal for Specialists in Group Work*, 38(1), 30–51.

Ohrt, J. H., Ener, E., Porter, J., & Young, T. L. (2014). Group leader reflections on their training and experience: Implications for group counselor educators and supervisors. *Journal for Specialists in Group Work*, 39(2), 95–124. doi:10.1080/01933922.2014.883004.

Pavey, L. & D. Donoghue (2003) The use of role play and VLEs in teaching environmental management. *Planet*, 10(1), 7–10. doi:10.11120/plan.2003.00100007.

Petty, G. (2006). *Evidence based teaching* (2nd ed.). Cheltenham: Nelson Thornes.

Rao, D. & Stupans, I. (2012). Exploring the potential of role play in higher education: development of a typology and teacher guidelines. *Innovations in Education and Teaching International*, 49 (4), 427–436.

Rosa, J.A. (2012). Marketing education for the next four billion: Challenges and innovations. *Journal of Marketing Education*, 34 (1), 44–54.

Rutan, S., W. Stone, & J. Shay (2014). *Psychodynamic Group Psychotherapy* (5th edition). New York: The Guilford Press.

Scheidlinger, S. (2004). Group interventions for treatment of trauma in children. In *Group Interventions for Psychological Trauma*. New York: American Group Psychotherapy Association.

Shapiro, L. & Leopold, J. (2012). A critical role for role-playing pedagogy. *TESL Canada Journal*, 29(2), 120–125. doi:10.18806/tesl.v29i2.1104.

Sogunro, O.A. (2004). Efficacy of role-playing pedagogy in training leaders: Some reflections. *Journal of Management Development*, 23(4), 355–371.

Steen, S., Vasserman-Stokes, E., & Vannatta, R. (2014). Group Cohesion in Experiential Growth Groups. *The Journal for Specialists in Group Work*, 39(3), 236–256.

Toriz, E. (2019). Learning based on flipped classroom with just-in-time teaching, UnityeD, gamification and educational spaces. *International Journal on Interactive Design and Manufacturing*, 13(3), 1159–1173. doi:10.1007/s12008-019-00560-z.

Walker, S. (2006). Journal writing as a teaching technique to promote reflection. *Journal of Athletic Training*, 41(2), 216–221.

Weiss, A. C., & Rutan, J. S. (2016). The benefits of group therapy observation for therapists-in-training. *International Journal of Group Psychotherapy*, 66(2), 246–260. doi:10.1080/00207284.2015.1111083.

Westrup, U. & Planander, A. (2013). Role-play as a pedagogical method to prepare students for practice: The students' voice. *Ogre utbildning*, 3(3), 199–210.

Woodbridge, L., & O'Beirne, B. (2017). Counseling Students' Perceptions of Journaling as a Tool for Developing Reflective Thinking. *The Journal of Counselor Preparation and Supervision*, 9(2).

Young, T. L., Reysen, R., Eskridge, T., & Ohrt, J. H. (2013). Personal growth groups: Measuring outcome and evaluating impact. *Journal for Specialists in Group Work*, 38(1), 52–67. doi:10.1080/01933922.2012.745915.

Zeide, E. (2019). Artificial Intelligence in higher education: Applications, promise and perils, and ethical questions. *Educause Review*, 54(3).

Ziomek-Daigle, J. (2017). Using Reflective Writing Practices to Articulate Student Learning in Counselor Education. *Journal of Creativity in Mental Health*, 12(2), 262–270.

3 Developing a Group Leader Therapeutic Self

The single most important component for successful group therapy is the group leader and the extent of their developed inner self (Yalom & Leszcz, 2021). It is not enough that the group leader learns skills and techniques, but they also will find it helpful to better understand how their selves influence and contribute to the growth, learning and healing for group members, and how it is their inner self that plays a major role for how and when to intervene.

The developed inner therapeutic self allows the group leader to be more effective as a group leader and to do the following.

- Better understand when and how to intervene.
- Identify and repair empathic failures.
- Effectively use objective countertransference to better understand what the group may be needing or find difficult to verbalize.
- Act as the group's container for intense/distressful feelings to better allow the member to be able to participate and manage their sensitive and uncomfortable feelings.
- Prevent and repair therapeutic ruptures that can affect the member(s) and the group as a whole.
- More effectively guide group members in self-exploration of unconscious material, unresolved issues that continue to impact their personal functioning, and other sensitive matters.
- Assist to form therapeutic alliances with individual members and with the group as a whole.
- Provide group process commentary about what the group is doing, not doing avoiding, and other unaware possibilities that are affecting the growth, development and healing for members and for the group.
- Understand member and group defenses, needs, and messages, which helps to formulate a group process comment.
- Manage difficult group members' behaviors without alienating them or producing fear for other group members.
- Constructively manage microaggressions and other insensitivities that have the potential for causing group ruptures and conflicts.

DOI: 10.4324/9781003329787-3

- Help develop trust and safety so that group members can disclose sensitive personal material, make meaningful connections among group members, and can more freely speak of their thoughts, feelings, and ideas in the here and now.
- Model effective relating and communication attitudes and behaviors that can help group members learn interpersonal skills that will be helpful in the group and in their lives.
- Recognize and foster the emergence of group therapeutic factors that are beneficial for the group members and for the group as a whole.
- Monitor potential harmful countertransference which occurs mainly on the unconscious level.

The Therapeutic Inner Self

The therapeutic self is a composite of self-awareness, self-reflection, the extent of understanding of personal psychological boundaries, identification of lingering family of origin issues and past unfinished business from previous relationships, as well as building a procedure for self-reflection and the constructive use of the leader's feelings in group session for intervention (s). These are useful as a foundation for implementing learned group facilitation skills, techniques and strategies.

Psychological Boundary Strength

Strong and resilient psychological boundary strength will aid the group leader to prevent emotional contagion and to resist projective identification. *Psychological boundary strength* helps to reduce emotional susceptibility and emotional contagion, and to prevent projective identification. Hatfield, Cacioppo, and Rapson (1993) describe the existence of emotional contagion, and how you may "catch" them when you are in the presence of people with intense emotions. This usually begins when someone silently and usually unconsciously "transmits" a feeling and the other person "catches" it. Sending and catching can be seen in the following examples.

- You interact with a depressed friend, and when you leave, you feel sad and despairing and this lasts for some time.
- You encounter a very happy person who talks to you about the event that produced the happiness and you find yourself smiling and your mood become more uplifting.

Projective identification is a form of emotional contagion. What happens is similar to the following. Think of when you were in an argument with someone. Both of you are angry, but the other person is much angrier than you are. However, as the argument continues, you find that your anger increased, and you decide to stop arguing and leave. As you walk away, you realize that your anger is or is almost rage, and you wonder how and why your anger got to this point. Even more troubling, you are not able to relinquish your feelings and the intensity does not lessen as it usually does in past similar situations. What happened is that the other person's emotions were sent (i.e. projected onto you), you caught them on top of those you were already experiencing, then you incorporated the projected emotions which then influenced how you felt.

Can *emotional contagion* be prevented? When the person's psychological boundaries are developed to be strong and resilient, they will be able to resist catching others' feelings. Working to develop psychological boundaries to be flexible and more under control is not only useful for preventing emotional contagion, developing strong and resilient psychological boundaries can also help in other ways. Examples include but are not limited to becoming less susceptible to being manipulated by others, achieving the ability to say no and stick to it, acting in one's best interests and not doing things that they don't want to do that someone else wants them to do, reduced feelings of being controlled by others, feeling that it is their responsibility to take care of others who are able to care for themselves, and an increased ability to tolerate others' distress without becoming enmeshed or overwhelmed. These are also examples of what can happen to the leader and to some group members in group therapy without conscious awareness.

Early Contributors to Development of the Inner Self

Among the many contributors to the development of the inner self are family of origin especially unresolved issues: aversive childhood experiences, cultural values, attitudes, and behaviors; unfinished business from past relationships; extent of self-absorption; and life experiences in general. Each person reacts and internalize these differently so that some have minimal influence and others are major contributors to the person that they become and many of these are not in conscious awareness. The leader's understanding of how these factors and experiences contributed to the person they became can help the leader to better understand what did or may have contributed to their group members' selves. A brief description of these contributors and their possible effects for the group leader follows.

Family of origin (FOO) experiences are the relationships that are developed with the parents, siblings, and other familial relationships that could affect the physical, cognitive, emotional and psychological development of the person. Yalom and Leszcz (2021) noted that the scripts developed in the family of origin are reenacted in the therapy group and this includes for the group leader also. Some of the FOO beliefs, attitudes and behaviors that were developed and can emerge in the group are the role in the family, how authority figures are perceived, transference, and the expression of feelings. Roles from family experiences for the group leader can be seen in the need to suppress or ignore conflict, a reluctance to challenge group members for fear of their disapproval, seeking admiration and approval from group members, and anxiety about their group leadership competence. An example of the impact of family of origin factors follows.

Vignette

> Bob, the group leader, grew up in a home where there was considerable conflict, particularly noisy fights between his parents almost every day. One or both parents would displace his/her anger and dissatisfaction on the children. Bob's brother and sister reacted by rebelling, and Bob became the "good" child who tried very hard to please his parents. As an adult, Bob valued harmony among people in his world, and would go to great lengths to achieve it.
>
> Bob was the leader of a group of young adults who were court-referred for Driving While under the Influence (DUI). He was uncomfortable from day one with the group because the three males in the group would verbally snipe at each other. When this happened, he would try to reframe the remark or redirect the topic. The group had met for 6 sessions and this night one of the women had joined the males in sniping at other members. Bob tried to stop it but that only resulted in all the group members getting angry or annoyed with him. Both Bob and the members left the group upset.

Analysis: Bob's need for harmony fueled his interventions and made him prone to jump in to try to defuse the situation rather than modeling how to constructively work through conflicts, and helping members learn how to express their thoughts and feelings. He seemed to take any hints of conflict personally, that is as being directed at him and were critical, or that he was supposed to do something about it. When a female group member joined in the sniping, old fears from his childhood where his parents fought emerged, and his reaction was predictable. He was more interested in getting his needs met that is, stopping the fight, than he was in the group needs. If he had been more confident, self-knowledgeable, and understanding of the group's needs that session, he would have re-directed the conflict between members to their real concern, such as dissatisfaction with the leader. He would have expected the attack because the group was in stage 2, and could have used it to show members that it was possible to express negative feelings and have positive results, neither the group, leader nor members would be destroyed, negative comments could be accepted without retaliation, members could express negative feelings and have them accepted and carefully considered, personal associations could be explored, they could learn how to constructively work through conflicts, understand how it is possible to not personalize negative comments, and thereby become narcissistically wounded.

Reflection: Some Important Family of Origin Experiences

Family of origin experiences are probably the most significant experiences that shaped an individual's development and are significant contributors to their values, perceptions of self and of others, and other factors that have influences on the self that the leader brings to the group. Parental conscious and unconscious messages, sibling relationships, traumatic events, and so on can continue to influence self-perceptions, relations with others, and provide material for countertransference in the group. Parental messages were received, incorporated into the developing self, acted on unconsciously, and are likely to continue to be major influences throughout life without conscious awareness. For example, old parental messages about the following may still be affecting you. Read these and reflect on how you may be still relating to and acting on these open and hidden messages.

- *Your value and worth as a person.*
- *Your looks, intellectual abilities, talents, and the like.*
- *The extent to which you were loved and cherished.*
- *Your parent's pleasure and admiration for you or the lack.*
- *How you were (are) to behave and relate to others.*
- *Unspoken parental expectations of and for you.*

These and other messages where how you learned early interpersonal relations, became acculturated to the family and to the community, and developed your self-perceptions. The responses, reactions, tolerance, acceptance, caring and concern you convey to group members are greatly influenced by these old parental messages. Many of these can be the basis for countertransference as the group leader.

Aversive childhood experiences are defined as abuse and/or neglect either physical, sexual or emotional, trauma, and as experiencing community and/or domestic violence. Aversive childhood experiences can lead to detrimental effects on psychological functioning, socialization, cognitive development, behavior problems, being hypervigilant, self-blame and a host of other negative outcomes and some may even continue to suffer from PTSD physical symptoms and effects. Adults who have had aversive childhood experiences can lack the awareness of the continuing impact of these on their relationships, emotional expression, and interpersonal interactions. Possible effects for AVE on the group leader can be seen in their use of self-criticism, fear of making mistakes so they don't intervene, suppression and avoidance of any hint of conflict, seeking attention and approval from group members, a refusal to admit mistakes, an inability to identify and repair empathic failures, and fears of being able to contain or manage members' intense emotions.

Cultural and diversity values, attitudes, and behaviors can be influential on the group leader without their conscious awareness. These are the elements that surround the person in their developing years that are transmitted to them by their family and community. The person absorbs the lessons about how to behave and relate, what is acceptable and not acceptable, what relationships to be developed, how to treat those that disagree, and many other relational aspects that will also be present in the group. It is important that the group leader maintain an awareness of how their culture plays a part in how they perceive and relate to group members as well as ensuring fair treatment. An awareness of different group members' values, attitudes and behaviors that may be the outcome of their cultural and diversity experiences can also play a role in the group leader's perceptions and relationships with group members. Some cultural and diversity influences are gender and sexual identities, religious beliefs, race/ethnic designations, age, educational levels, occupation, country/region, language, and many other factors. These can play out in the group also and affect how the therapeutic relationship is affected, unconscious or nonconscious unfair or unequal treatment of group members, an unawareness of members' transference, misunderstanding emotional expressions, and other such important factors.

Unfinished business from past relationships can also be influential. Much of our self-development is formed by others' perceptions and behaviors to us, and all of the relationships we have throughout life can carry some unfinished business – a gestalt therapy term to indicate that past relationships can continue to affect the person's well-being. Unfinished business means that other relationships helped form current self-perceptions and behaviors that may be affecting self-esteem, ability to form and maintain enduring and satisfying relationships, produce caution and wariness about trying to form new relationships, countertransference which is unconscious for the leader by definition, and other self and relational factors. The group leader can unintentionally erect barriers to defend against some group members because of this unfinished business, or fail to take some actions such as intervening with difficult member behaviors, or failing to maintain group boundaries and rules.

Extent of adult self-absorption are those behaviors and attitudes that are reflective of undeveloped, stable (Kohut, 1977) or destructive (Brown, 2021) narcissism which is not seen by the person. While not necessarily diagnosable as narcissism, self-absorption can reflect some on those behaviors and attitudes although to a lesser intensity and extent. Self-absorption is conceptualized as being on a continuum that includes pathological (NPD), destructive, stable and heathy adult. The next section addresses how to reduce self-absorption.

Reduce Self-Absorption

Presented here are some descriptors for behavior and attitudes that are reflective of self-absorption for the leader and the possible effects on group members. The descriptors are grandiosity, entitlement, lack of empathy, attention needs, admiration needs, exploitation of others, extensions of self, shallow emotions, the impoverished ego, emptiness, unique and special and envy. Most of these are not in conscious awareness but can be seen by others.

Grandiosity is an inflated self where they are all powerful and others are expected to recognize this characteristic. Excessive grandiosity seen in a group leader could include pushing a member to disclose more than they want to, telling members what they should or ought to be and do, having to be the "expert" on just about everything, and never admitting a mistake. *Entitlement* is the expectation that the person can do whatever they want to do without objections from others. Conveys a superior attitude, and more time and effort is spent on meeting the leader's needs. Group members can feel shamed, guilty, and inadequate. *Lack of empathy* shows an indifference to others' concerns and feelings. Group members can feel diminished, devalued or discounted and unworthy when their feelings are ignored, overlooked or passed over.

Attention needs of the leader leads to the group becoming more about the leader and their need to be the center of attention than about the group members. *Admiration needs* of the leader become central for the members, and considerable group time is spent on ingratiation and saying and doing things that support the leader's need to be admired. *Exploitation of others* occurs when the leader uses members to meet their needs rather than helping the group members and the group to meet their needs. Members can feel manipulated, taken advantage of and not respected.

Extensions of self occurs when there is an incomplete understanding of where one ends, and where others begin and can be seen in group leader's actions such as insisting that members disclose shameful material, trying to "break down resistance", and in seeking "breakthroughs".

Shallow emotions in the group leader affects group members because of the lack of modeling for experiencing and expressing a range and variety of emotions. In addition, the leader may set the norm that only certain emotions, such as anger and fear, are appropriate for expressing in the group. *Impoverished ego* is the flip side of grandiosity and coexists with it. The impoverished self is the self that is constantly seeking for reassurance of worthiness, presents the self as of little value and in constant danger of being destroyed, and is very anxious with the expectation that others exist to take care of them. This state can be seen in group leaders who expect the group members to meet their needs, such as their need or expectation for participation, and become hurt when this fails to happen. *Emptiness* within is not numbness, loneliness or depression but is a sense that the person has that their lives are lacking meaning and purpose. They are not deriving pleasure and joy for their lives and feel that they are missing what others have. *Unique and special* can also be a sign of feelings of entitlement and superiority. The person wants and expects deference, expect others to obey their commands, and demanding of special recognition. Group members can come to feel that they are fatally flawed, extremely inadequate, and unworthy. *Envy* is the conviction that someone else is undeserving and unworthy of what they accomplish or have, and that the envious person is much more deserving.

Some leader thoughts that can signal self-absorption are the following. Each is explained in a later section in this chapter.

- Do they like me?
- They won't like me if I _____ .
- Am I doing it right?
- They are being so (stubborn, resistant, defensive, unfair).
- Why aren't they cooperating?
- I'm doing the best that I can.
- I want (need) the group to think that I'm (good/expert/competent/likeable).
- What can I do that will please them?
- They should ...
- They ought to ...
- They are so unappreciative.

Reducing or eliminating the leader's self-absorption is essential for preventing negative effects on the group and/or group members.

Negative Effects of Leader Self-Absorption on the Group

The leader who has considerable self-absorbed behaviors and attitudes can have a negative effect on the group and on the members. Included but not limited to the more destructive effects are indecisiveness, arrogance, vindictiveness, pushing members for disclosures, the possible harm for unconscious countertransference, and favoritism.

Indecisiveness displayed by the group leader is very anxiety producing for group members. The impoverished ego state of having to not make a mistake, or that the leader is more concerned about how they come across to group members can lead to indecisiveness for the group leader.

Arrogance can be exhibited when the group leader is overly confident which is conveying that the leader is superiority, can lead to taking risks where group members may be harmed, and are more focused on the group leader's needs that for those of the group.

Vindictiveness can be seen when the group leader engages in behaviors that produce shame and feelings of inadequacy for group members. Pushing members to disclose more than they want to, and other manipulative and exploitative behaviors.

Pushing for deeper self-disclosure is not being respectful of group members' abilities to make personal decisions about when and how much they want to disclose. While the group leader may be able to build some trust and safety for group members, not all group members may achieve this feeling of safety and are more cautious about personal disclosures.

Unawareness of personal subjective countertransference as defined by Yalom and Leszcz (2021) occurs from the influence of past negative experiences and relationships on current relationships.

Examples for leaders' subjective countertransference include but are not limited to the following. Having a strong like or dislike for one or more group members, ignoring or minimizing conflict among group members or with the leader, not identifying or repairing many empathic failures, becoming deeply wounded or angry when members are critical, telling, demanding or even thinking how a member should or ought to think, or react, or behave, and/or becoming exasperated, irritated, annoyed, or angry with a group member or members.

Favoritism occurs when the leader favors or seems to favor a group member by giving them more attention, approval, and agreement, while others are ignored, dismissed, or received in an indifferent manner.

Understand How Personal Issues Influence Thoughts and Feelings

Some indices of leader self-absorption were presented earlier under the section titled "Contributors" and following are explanations of how these thoughts and feelings can lead to ineffective leader interventions and can lead to attacks on the leader. Let's explore how and why these have an impact.

"*Do they like me?*" is just another way to express a deep need for liking and approval. An individual who has a need like this can be deeply hurt if someone does or says anything that hints of dislike or disapproval. He/she will go out of their way to gain others' liking and approval, even to the point of not behaving wisely. It is desirable, but not essential, that the group leader be liked by group members. What is essential is that the group leader be trusted and respected, and that is unlikely to occur if members feel that you can be manipulated to gain their liking and approval. Members will like you if you "are" the kind of person who is caring, and can attend to their safety needs.

"*Am I doing it right?*" also speaks of the need for approval but could also be reflective of a mind-set such as, "if I do this, then that will occur". If–then thinking is not yet applicable to group counseling as the dynamics of the group, and its members are unique for each group. It is not possible to accurately predict what will happen for anything you do or say. The need to "do it right" assumes that there is a "right" way and, that you are inadequate or flawed if you don't do what is right. Again, the focus is on you rather than the group and its members.

"*Why are they resisting?*" is a thought that carries an implication that members should not have resistance. It also implies that you think that you should do something and/or that you did something to cause the resistance. It's all about you, not about group members. It is much more constructive to note where there is resistance, what seemed to trigger it, and what defense mechanism is used. You do not have to "do" anything. In fact, it's best if you do not do anything. If the group as a whole is resisting, you would be more constructive if you would turn your thinking to analyzing what the group is trying to tell you by the resistance. The group may be saying:

- "This doesn't address our need."
- "It doesn't feel safe."

- "This is too scary (sensitive, etc.)."
- "We are afraid of being hurt."
- "You are meeting your need – not ours."

These are some of the negative impact and effects that the group and members may encounter. Instead of being guided for growth, development, and healing, they are being made to feel inadequate, guilty, shames and not valued as a worthwhile unique individual.

Self-reflection

Self-reflection can be of enormous benefit for the group leader as this process has been show to reduce stress (Gale & Schroder, 2014), aid in case formulation, and to help monitor the possibility of countertransference. Group leaders can also increase their awareness of their leadership strengths and weaknesses and for the interventions they choose to employ. This focus on the self for reviewing the session and/or the progress of the group allows the group leader to better identify how their actions are benefiting the group and the members, to allow recognition of possible empathic failures, to reinforce what they are doing that is beneficial, and to explore their reactions in the group for possible countertransference.

Bennett-Levy et al. (2009) defines self-reflection as a conscious understanding of one's emotions, thoughts and attitudes when they occurred so as to gather more information about what is being done and said, and possible underlying rationales for these. In other words, while some of what is being experienced can be on the nonconscious or unconscious levels, these can become more visible and apparent when reflected on so as to either capitalize on them, or to prevent their potentially harmful effects. An illustrative example that happened to one of my students was when he very much wanted to comment on a social justice issue that emerged in the group session because that topic was intensely important to him. The group members were actively engaged in the discussion and were voicing their opinions and perspective. He reported that he tried to quickly reflect in that moment as to why he felt the need to comment, and realized that it was a reflection of some possible countertransference, and reminded himself that the group members were carrying the discussion.

To monitor possible countertransference during or even after a session, the group leader can reflect on the following.

- "What am I feeling, or aware of right now?"
- "I am feeling _____."
- "What happened that seemed to trigger this response or feeling?"
- "Did the exchange, event, interaction, etc., hold the potential for my personal projections, etc.?"
- "Could it be that what I am experiencing is countertransference?"

- "What are my personal associations for the triggering event?"
- "To this point I don't think what I am experiencing is due to my personal issues. What other possibilities are there?"
- "Would it be helpful to the group to openly speak of my experiencing, relate my feelings, etc.?"
- "Is it possible that I am containing some unspoken feelings for the group?"

These can be guides for understanding the group's process and as a prevention for possible therapeutic ruptures or even harm.

A self-reflective stance has both a personal growth outcome and is a group leader skill and technique. This is one way of building self-understanding and the inner therapeutic self. But, it is also a valuable tool for understanding what is taking place in the group, what is important for the group, what is crucial for the group, and what is a concern for its members. Knowing what the group needs and what to do or how to intervene becomes easier with a self-reflective stance.

However, care should be taken so that the leader's self-reflection does not result in destructive forces for the group and/or its members. Destructive forces include countertransference, meeting the leader's personal needs, self-absorption, emotionally distancing from the group, retreat from conflict or intense feelings, minimizing members' concerns, withdrawal of support, and/or failure to be empathic or appropriately intervene. You may wonder how any of these relate to your expertise as a group leader. The clinical vignette about Bob presented earlier in the chapter is an example of what is meant.

It is highly possible that Bob had participated in counseling or therapy but had not completely worked through some personal family of origin issues. Thus, when faced with a situation that tapped into his personal issues, he reacted on the basis of his personal needs. It is much more beneficial for the leader to explore and work on his personal issues outside the group. Working with a therapist is the most effective way to become aware of personal issues, especially family of origin issues. However, personal growth can take place in other ways, and can enhance therapy.

Self-reflection can be helpful in other ways. One especially important assistance it can provide is when the leader is attacked. At some point the group will likely mount an attack on the group leader. The attack may be mild, indirect, or open and direct. This is an expected behavior in stage two and is perceived as a positive event for group progress. The group leader who fears attacks and works to keep the group from attacking them, is not helping members to learn how to manage, contain, and appropriately express aggressive, hostile, and destructive feelings. The leader who has a strong need for liking and approval can be hurt when the attack occurs, and not react in a constructive way. This leader can think, "Why are they (the group members) so stubborn/unfair/defensive?", or "Why aren't they cooperating?", or "I'm doing the best I can". These are not constructive thoughts as they are all focused on the leader, and their thoughts and feelings. The leader is more concerned about their personal feelings and is blaming and criticizing members for arousing the feelings instead of focusing on the group, its needs, and what members are trying to communicate via the attack. It is much more helpful for the group leader to use the personal feeling aroused as a guide to understanding what members are feeling and trying to communicate.

For example, suppose you are the group leader, and members have been cooperative and participating for the first four sessions. You are expecting the same behavior for the fifth session and have planned what to do and say to move the group toward a goal. However, shortly after the session begins, members begin making comments, and asking questions that are arousing irritation and mild resentment in you. One member in particular continues to press you for answers you feel you have already provided. Another member interrupts you to ask what are they supposed to be doing, and how is this supposed to help. You begin to wonder what is happening, and your feelings of irritation and resentment are joined by feelings of inadequacy, incompetence, and uncertainty.

A constructive use of these feelings would be to focus on the group, and its message. The underlying message could be that members are getting in touch with their personal feelings of being flawed and are irritated at you for putting them in a position where they cannot escape experiencing them and are expected to examine these uncomfortable feelings. They are uncomfortable and are blaming the leader for their discomfort. Once you reach this point in understanding of what the group may be experiencing, a response could be to acknowledge their feelings with something like, "It's not easy to do this work and experience the uncomfortable feelings that are aroused". Another response could an acknowledgement of their irritation with you, such as saying, "You are irritated that I am doing and saying things that trigger uncomfortable feelings for you, and you wonder how that is supposed to help you."

Not only could self-reflection suggest positive interventions, but it could also help to prevent unconstructive interventions such as responding with any of the following.

- "The group seems really hostile today."
- "Let's work on your goals."
- "We're here to work on your problems and I'm trying to help you."
- "What happened to make you so cranky today?"
- "What do you want to talk about?"
- "I've tried to answer your questions, but nothing seems to satisfy you."

None of the above responses would acknowledge the message from the group or that the leader would carefully consider that message.

It is also helpful to use *self-reflection during sessions*. Self-reflection can be of enormous benefit when leading a group. Leaders will have to develop their own style and expertise to both tune in to their inner experiencing, and to what the group and its members are doing and saying simultaneously. This is not easy to do trying to tune in to inner experiencing while at the same time observe what is happening in the group as the focus on one can less attention to the other. It can be easy to get lost in personal thoughts or be consumed by what members are doing and saying. Of most importance is the extent to which you can trust what you are experiencing to recognize group level process, identify members' feelings, understand the "real message", make empathic responses, decide on the best response or intervention, tap into resistance and sensitive areas, and identify empathic failures. As noted before, when you can trust what emerges for you personally, you can identify what is needed and know better what can be effective responses and interventions.

Group leaders who want to use the resources of the group to help individual members will make constructive use of group level process commentary. There are times when your inner experiencing is a vital clue to what is taking place in the group and is the basis for process commentary. It can also provide information about the relationship between the leader and a member. Hence, the ability to tap into personal experiencing can help which gaining an understanding of what is wanted, needed, desired, and so on, on a much deeper level by the group and/or member. This use of self-reflection is immediate, quick, capable of mirroring, and uses both thoughts and feelings. These are but a few examples of the constructive use for self-reflection in the group and with members.

The leader's responding has to be immediate as they do not have time to engage in considerable or considered self-reflection. There is a time and place or need for that of course, but not during the session. This use of self-reflection demands that the leader stay present centered with the group while engaging in self-reflection. Thus, the leader has to be confident that the feelings they experience at that time are not reflective of their unresolved issues, biases, transference, etc., but are an accurate reflection of what is taking place in the group or with a member.

The response must also be quick in the sense that the leader does not wait until later in the session before deciding what to say or do. Sometimes they may do nothing because that is the best response. What the leader does not want to happen is that they do nothing because they are paralyzed or completely ignorant of what to do. Responding later in the session is better than not responding at all. However, learning to quickly engage in self-reflection and make appropriate responses at that optimum time is a skill to learned and practiced.

When a group leader becomes aware of what feelings are clearly personal, when projective identification occurs and/or, when they may be acting as the container for the group's feelings, that will suggest the intervention.

If for example, the intervention is to mirror the particular feeling for the person and/or the group that can be very helpful if acting as the container for the group's feeling. For example, when all or most, group members are anxious and fearful, but refuse to accept their feelings or try to suppress or deny them, and the leader finds that they are becoming increasingly anxious that could signal that the leader may be acting as the "container" for the group's feelings. The group members project their feelings, the leader incorporates the feelings so that members do not have to experience them, and the leader is then containing the members' unpleasant feelings. If the leader can realize what is happening and mirror these feelings to the group, get members to accept and acknowledge their feelings, then the leader can cease being the container and members have learned to manage their anxiety.

It is helpful to be able to use both thoughts and feelings during your self-reflection. Thoughts will help you analyze and stay connected to objective reality while, at the same time, use the valuable and probably accurate information from your feelings. It's best not to rely solely on either as being truthful, real, accurate, better, and so on, it's best to use both.

When the leader acts on what they perceive is happening in the group or with a member, they may also be tapping their inner wisdom. This use of self-reflection is helpful to the group when there is an impasse; a continuing conflict or reemergence of a conflict that was thought to be resolved; nothing seems to be taking place in the group; prolonged silence; there is inability to stay focused; members engage in considerable chit-chat; the emphasis is on there and then topics; and/or expression of intense affect is ignored.

Self-reflection is helpful for working with individual members when a member is doing any of the following.

- Exhibiting dependence on the leader, lobbying for the leader's approval, and/or becoming more needy.
- Challenges the leader instead of expressing their feelings. This is one way members can avoid acceptance of their feelings or other material that is potentially dangerous.
- Engaging in problem behaviors such as monopolizing, withdrawing, initiating discord, and the like.
- Your responses and comments appear to be off-target, or unacceptable to a member. The yes–but member response is another example.
- A member is trying to express their experiencing but cannot verbalize it and the leader can assist with their expression.
- A member is hostile, aggressive, combative, and initiates some conflict or discord.

Self-reflection by the leader could help to suggest an effective intervention.

Emotional Presence

One important component for an inner therapeutic self is emotional presence in interactions. The leader's emotional presence has many benefits for the group that involve the following; provide clues for group as a whole factors, prevent therapeutic ruptures, tune into members' distress, help to suggest when and how to intervene, more easily identify empathic failures so that they can be repaired quicker, and act as a model for positive interpersonal interactions (Geller & Greenberg, 2012; Geller, Greenberg, & Watson, 2010; Geller, Pos, & Colosimo, 2012; Geller & Porges, 2014; Pawrelczyk, 2019).

Emotional presence also referred to in some publications as "presence in psychotherapy" for the group leader is very important for a number of reasons that include the following.

Members can feel that the leader *hears and understands* what they are trying to convey which can lead to a corrective emotional experience, will help to build trust and safety among the group members, and is encouraging and supportive of additional member's disclosures. Emotional presence is very helpful to promote the ability to tune into *group level process* and other group as a whole factors. *Nonverbal communications* can be more readily observed and understood when the leader is emotionally present. It is easier to identify empathic failures so that these can be repaired in the here and now. *Group level and individual resistance* is more readily identified when the group leader can tune into their current experiencing when observing the group.

Observation of the presence or absence of *group therapeutic factors* can help with identification of these and suggest interventions to help their emergence in the group. The group leader is more able to *act as a container* for members' feelings which can help members to be freer to express these and not become mired in them.

The emotionally present group leader is able to screen or block out distractions, intrusive thoughts especially those about personal concerns, and to bring their full attention to the here and now of the group. Just maintaining eye contact is not sufficient as some group members are able to discern when the "self" of the group leader is present or absent. This is not something that can be taught and learned as cognitive or even experiential material, it has to be a part of the person and intentional for the benefit of the group and its members.

An emotional presence in the session requires that the group leader first be aware of and manage their personal anxiety and to bring their attention to the here and now. During the group session, it is helpful for the group leader to look at the group and individual members, listen for content and feelings as well as for what seems to be avoided or ignored, try to feel what emotions members are expressing and/or feeling, and to try to stay open and available for taking in some intangibles such as resistance, transference, intensity of feelings expressed or unexpressed, and other group factors.

Additional Learning

This chapter presented a rationale, explanation, and examples for some elements of a therapeutic self. Illustrations for how these elements could affect the group and its members were described as well as suggestions for developing these elements. Harder to address will be the unconscious effects for family of origin and other experiences, the impact of some undeveloped self-absorption, and other personal development. Examples and suggestions were given for applications to some commonly occurring group situations and events.

Although most of the remaining chapters will focus on knowledge factors, techniques, and strategies, there will also be references to the therapeutic self. Some knowledge, techniques, and strategies will be more effective with the addition of the therapeutic self and what is presented about the therapeutic self can also be used to better understand group members and well as some group as a whole factors and concepts.

References

Bennett-Levy, J. & Perry, H. (2009). The promise of online cognitive behavioral therapy training for rural and remote mental health professionals. *Australasian Psychiatry*, 17(suppl.), S121–S124. doi:10.1080/10398560902948126.

Brown, N. (2018). *Psychoeducational Groups* (4th edition). New York: Routledge.

Brown, N. (2021). *Understanding Narcissists*. Santa Barbara, CA: ABC-CLIO/Praeger.

Gale, C. & Schroder, T. (2014). Experiences of self-practice/self-reflection in cognitive behavioural therapy: a meta-synthesis of qualitative studies. *Psychological Psychotherapy* 87(4), 373–392. doi:10.1111/papt.12026.

Geller, S., & Greenberg, L. (2012). *Therapeutic Presence: A Mindful Approach to Effective Therapy*. Washington, DC: American Psychological Association.

Geller, S., Greenberg, L., & Watson, J. C. (2010). Therapist and client perceptions of therapeutic presence: The development of a measure. *Psychotherapy Research*, 20(5), 599–610.

Geller, S., & Porges, S. W. (2014). Therapeutic presence: Neurophysiological mechanisms mediating feeling safe in therapeutic relationships. *Journal of Psychotherapy Integration*, 24(3), 178.

Geller, S., Pos, A., & Colosimo, K. (2012). Therapeutic presence: A common factor in the provision of effective psychotherapy. *Society for Psychotherapy Integration*, 47, 6–13.

Hatfield, E., Cacioppo, J., & Rapson, R. (1993). *Emotional Contagion*. Cambridge: Cambridge University Press.

Kohut, H. (1977). *The restoration of the self*. Madison, CT: International Universities.

Pawrelczyk, J. (2019). The therapist emotional presence and its interactional functions in promoting client change in relationship-focused integrative psychotherapy. *Communication and Medicine*, 16(2). doi:10.1558/cam.33823.

Stone, W. (2017). Self-psychology: Empathy and process. *International Journal of Group Psychotherapy*, 67(1), 164–170.

Yalom, I. & Leszcz, M. (2021). *The Theory and Practice of Group Psychotherapy* (6th edition). New York: Basic Books.

4 Organizing and Structuring the Group

General Guidelines for Planning

Let's start with a reflection about a previous group experience, either one where you were a member or one that you were the leader.

Activity: Group Reflection and Image

Materials: It will be helpful if you can write your responses to the activity and keep it where it is easily assessable. Paper and a writing instrument are used.

Directions: Sit in a quiet place, close your eyes if you like and visualize a group that you were the leader. It does not matter what type of group: any group leadership experience will suffice.

1   Write a short description of the group as you remember it noting the feelings you had then and are not aware of about that group.
2   Now, write a brief paragraph about your planning for that group and how that helped or hindered your group facilitation. Identify and write the most positive experience(s) associated with this group, the most negative experience(s), what you did as the leader that was most effective, what you did that was least effective, what you think or wish that you had planned or done differently.
3   Describe how better planning could have been helpful.

Planning and assessment are critical and essential for effective groups and are the responsibility of the group leader, even when the group is a repeat of groups that you have facilitated in the past. The discussion on planning is divided into four sections: Pre-group considerations, a model for planning a group, a sample plan, and assessment.

Pre-group Considerations

There are several pre-group considerations to think about prior to planning a particular group: the group leader's training and scope of practice,

DOI: 10.4324/9781003329787-4

research findings about the group's focus, the extent of the group leader's authority and responsibility and relevant members' characteristics.

The group leader's training and scope of practice is essential to consider when planning a group. While the basics usually achieved in training is usually sufficient, the potential group leader must have had didactic and experiential training that included group level facilitative skills, the conditions and group treatment planning. A major pre-planning activity is to *research findings about the condition, issue or concern* that will be the focus for the group (Kalodner & Coughlin, 2004). New information is being released all of the time, and there may be more to be learned and could be helpful for the group and its members.

Group leaders will find it helpful to establish the *extent of their authority and responsibility* prior to and as a part of the planning process. Leaders of many groups will not be able to select group members, or to screen out people who may be unsuitable, as the membership may be predetermined and participants ordered or forced to attend group therapy. Knowing *relevant members' characteristics* can be a critical component and although it may not be possible to know some of the vital information in advance, it is still important to know some of the members' characteristics so as to better plan the group to be relevant. Essential member information includes educational levels, present condition, medication effects, presence of past traumas, and if the members will be voluntary or mandated.

Educational levels of group members can be a significant factor to know in advance to ensure that members will understand what is being presented. Members' *present condition* or illnesses play a role for their participation in the group, what can be taught and learned, and other things such as selection of appropriate activities. Leaders should be familiar with the various effects the conditions or illnesses can have on the member(s) and pay particular attention on the attention span that can be expected; the extent of cognitive functioning or impairment, the effect on affective functioning and expression such as mood swings, and inappropriate expressions of feelings; effects on relationships and so on. The *effects of medication(s)* can also be important to know or research in advance as these may impair members' attention, participation, and learning. Sedating effects, or their lack when prescribed medication is not taken, stimulating effects that produce hyperactivity, and lack of pain reduction are some effects that can impact members' participation, interactions, and learning. Some members may have more than one condition or illness, or there can be another associated illness or condition in addition to the major or presenting one. Significant *past traumas* can be of vital importance in planning to help the group leader to better prepare for members' reactions and participation, the selection of activities and other experiences, and the possibility of these to trigger old memories, especially when these were not resolved earlier. Group leaders can be better prepared if they know in advance whether the members are attending *voluntarily or if they are mandated* to attend. Group dynamics and factors such as resistance, willingness to participate and disclose, and openness to learning are some of the members' group involvement that can be affected by mandated attendance.

Group Characteristics, Screening, and Orientation

Pre-planning incorporates knowing if the group is to be *open or closed* where new members are constantly added, or a *closed group* where no new members are added after the group begins. The *setting for the group* such as being inpatient, residential, outpatient, or for an institution such as a school or university will affect this structure.

It is recommended that potential group members be *screened* for appropriateness for the group as there are individuals who will not benefit from participation. Some criteria for exclusion presented by MacNair-Semands and Lese (2000) include current and significant substance abuse, impaired cognitive functioning, active psychosis, extensive social inhibition, and extreme anger or hostility. Criteria for inclusion can include the ability to actively participate in group, level of commitment to change, the capacity for self-reflection, and acceptable interpersonal relating and communication skills (Gans & Alonso, 1998). It is also recommended that members receive a pre-group *orientation* which allows the group leader to describe what the group is about, the expectations of group members, help the prospective member set realistic goals for their participation, and to answer questions and concerns that they may have. Orientation can take place during screening or at the first group session.

It is best when the group leader can screen prospective group members and when they orient the members to the group. Many times, the group leader may not be able to screen members for suitability for group therapy as the agency or the like requires clients to participate in groups. However, it is possible for group leaders to provide members with orientation to the group if not in a pre-group session, then during the first session of the group.

Screening of potential group members is of considerable help when planning the group as this allows the group leader to estimate the need for protection of the member and for the group. The screening process can provide information about the group member's language facility, expectations and hopes for benefits from the group experience, fears about the group and the leader, personal cultural and diversity needs, fears about emotional/issue/concerns contagion, barriers to participation such as a disability that would prevent or hinder participation in art activities, level of commitment to personal change and growth, emotional control and regulation, and other factors that will play a role for the member's participation and potential for growth. Protection for the group may be determined from information gathered from and about prospective group members during screening that may negatively impact the group and/or other members. Information gathered can allow the group leader to judge the suitability of the person for the proposed group, the mix of group members, and any personal negative attitudes, prejudices, biases, and/or other cultural and diversity characteristics that may affect acceptance by and of others, and participation.

Screening and selection of potential group members are important due to the intimate nature of groups, the intensity of feelings that will be explored, the personal disclosures that will be shared, and the need for members to respect and care for each other. Safety and trust are critical for group members and a process of screening and selection can provide some information to the group leader about how potential members will fit in, interact, and profit from the group experience.

The American Group Psychotherapy Association's Best Practice Guidelines (AGPA & IBCGP, 2002) emphasize the importance of *pre-group preparation* and provide evidence for its efficacy. Pre-group preparation includes informing members about expected behaviors in group, the aims of the group, and the techniques and processes the leader will use. Orientation to the group can help members develop personal goals which will later be integrated with group goals, reduce some of their anxiety about the uncertain and unknown, and start to set the foundation for establishing the therapeutic alliance.

The two most important decisions for the group leader are the suitability of the person for the group experience, and the possible fit with the group (AGPA & IBCGP, 2002). The personal member characteristics most closely associated with positive results for group therapy include high motivation), their attraction and commitment to the group work), interpersonal competency, and the value and desire for personal change.

It is the group leader's subjective judgment that determines whether the person is a possible good fit for the group. The guiding principles for selection are the extent to which their personal goals mesh with the group goals, do they have realistic and realistic expectations for changes, and can a viable therapeutic alliance be established.

Components for Planning Groups

The structural components for planning groups include the target audience, purpose and goals, when and where sessions will be held, planned treatment, and assessment. Basic components for the target audience include if the group is open or closed, screening and selection of group members, group size, if the group will have homogeneous/heterogeneous, membership, members' educational level(s), ages, gender identity, occupation, country of origin, and if they are voluntary or involuntary group participants, and their present condition.

Educational level is an important consideration for adult groups because it plays a role in the leader's decisions about what information to present, instructional strategies, and the amount of information that can be absorbed and learned. Then too, there can be members' apprehensions about being included or excluded because of their educational level. Mixing a wide range of educational levels can sometimes produce a rich experience, but sometimes it can make for a difficult and uncomfortable group experience because of members' fears, defensiveness, or arrogance. *Gender identity* is a factor that can produce considerable projection, transference, apprehension, and possible eroticism in groups. Members' previous experiences, expectations for behaviors and attitudes are some of the aspects that may trigger projections, transference and other reactions.

Decide if the group will have *homogeneous or heterogeneous membership.* Homogeneous groups where members have many important characteristics in common generally can more easily develop safety and trust because of perceived similarities. However, these groups can get so caught up in the desire and need to maintain harmony, that conflicts and the like are ignored or suppressed. Heterogeneous groups that have a mixture of members with important characteristics will have more perceived differences among members and those differences can contribute to some positive aspects such as a variety of perspectives and experiences but, can also have some restraining factors such as members being tentative and wary in the beginning, of the group and safety and trust may take longer to develop. However, heterogeneous groups can have a richness of resources because of the diversity. Regardless of the differences, these groups can become cohesive around shared important commonalties.

Location concerns refer to the size and comfort of the room (space) where the group meets, intrusions and disruptions are eliminated or minimized, and there is adequate equipment available if needed. Setting the frame for the group includes determining the *purpose, goal(s), objectives* (learning and affective), and *proposed leader strategies.* The purpose for the group is usually an identified a deficiency, lack of information, a needed upgrade or development of skills that would increase efficiency and productivity, and so on. The leader's tasks are to develop preliminary goals and objectives, and during the first session they invite members to accept or reject or modify these, and also ask if there are other goals that members want included. It is also helpful in advance to develop a set of rules and expectations for members' behaviors, select specific strategies and activities, specify what is planned to occur, and to gather materials and supplies.

Goals are expected or desired end outcomes for participation in the group, and should be defined as such, be measurable or observable, and are realistic for the expected group experience. Keep the number of goals to one or two. *Objectives* are steps or processes used to attain the goals and can focus on more specific behavior that is also measurable and/or observable. These should be stated in terms of what members will be able to do as a result of participating in the group. Once the goals and objectives are developed and written, group leaders can better select strategies that are designed to help meet the goals and objectives.

Burlingame et al. (2011) propose that group leaders define the *group rules* and communicate these to members. Brown (2003) suggests that the number of rules be kept small and focused on the behaviors necessary for keeping order in the group. Rules that may be common for all groups are attendance expectations, use of electronic devices, refrain from physically aggressive behavior, that respect, civility, and courtesy shall be shown to other members and to the leader, and no smoking, alcohol or illegal drug use or influence. The type of group may direct the development of rules for that group.

Another component for the group's frame is to determine in advance the *number of sessions*, how *long each session* will meet, and *how often* sessions will be held. Components for sessions such as activities, lectures, and other treatment planning are also determined in advance. Finally, it is important to have a plan to assess the efficacy of the group, the components, the leadership, and outcomes.

It is recommended that group leaders write a plan for each session. Plans are flexible and can be modified as the group unfolds, but it is helpful to start with a plan for how each session will be connected to the goals and objectives, the strategies that will be used, what equipment may be needed, and the material and supplies to be used.

Children's Groups

Critical components when planning for children's groups are their ages, educational level, and the purpose for the group. Group leaders should be prepared to fully describe orally and in writing what is planned for the group, to present this to both the children and their parents for obtaining informed consent which must be obtained before the group begins.

Try to limit the range of ages and educational levels in a group, and do not mix too many different ages or educational levels. Other organizing elements include: a limited range of ages, planning for briefer sessions, selecting instructional strategies and activities that take into account members' attention spans, using more active experiences, building groups and/or sessions around themes, and limiting information.

Adolescent Groups

Some basic considerations for leading adolescent groups include length of sessions, span of ages in the group, containing and managing intense emotions, and the need for structuring and directing. *Containing and managing intense emotions* for almost all adolescents are leader tasks that should be expected. The leader's skill at containing and managing these provides the space where the group members can explore issues and concerns in the session, teaches them that emotions can be managed, and provides modeling of how that is accomplished. There is a considerable need for *structure and direction* to help adolescents know what the limits are, to let them understand that safety is recognized as important, to emphasize the group's purpose and goals, and to give support for helping to contain and manage anxiety. It may be advisable to have a set of procedures for each session, and to stick to this as much as possible.

Adult and Older Adult Groups

In addition to the previous general guidelines, some other significant factors for adult and older adult groups can be cognitive abilities and educational level, gender, and current support system. Adults and older adult group members may have differing *cognitive abilities*. It can be helpful for leaders to know and stay aware of the possible effects of members' cognitive ability as this can significantly impact learning, understanding, and interactions in the group. Central to fostering hope and recovery is the extent of a *member's support system*. Although this factor is outside the group, it can be helpful for members to become aware of the strengths and weaknesses of their support system, to begin to develop and/or strengthen it, and to capitalize on this resource.

Assessment and Evaluation

Much valuable information can be gathered from assessment that can be used to determine the efficacy of the group, evaluate the members' progress and their satisfaction with the group experience, and positive and negative aspects of leadership. An ideal assessment plan begins with a focus on the goals and objectives for the group, and to evaluate if and how these were accomplished or not accomplished. Therefore, it is critical that these be phrased in a way that allows for assessment and stated in behavioral terms such as what the group members will be able to do at the end of the group. It is helpful to state these using terms such as list, define, describe, and demonstrate which allows for more objective evaluation or appraisal of accomplishment.

The efficacy of the group refers to the extent to which the goals and objectives were met. When goals and objectives are written in advance in behavioral terms, then they can be more easily assessed after the group ends. *Evaluating members' progress* relies on the pre-planning definitions for progress and/or success. Written in behavioral terms makes it easier to evaluate the extent to which members met their personal goals and the group's goals.

Evaluating strategies used in group sessions. Every group uses several strategies and/or materials, and it is helpful to gain information about the effectiveness and efficacy of those used for the group. This information will be helpful for the planning for future groups. Members can evaluate materials about the impact readability, and general helpfulness of materials. This information can lead to refinement of choices for materials and, in some cases, refinement of the materials. *Evaluation of environmental factors* include the physical comfort of facilities, privacy the room afforded, the extent to which disruptions were eliminated or minimized and so on. The vast majority of groups that have any assessment at all use participants' opinions to *evaluate the group leader.* This can be used to gather information about any changes in members' functioning coping and attitudes in addition to members' reactions to materials, instruction, leadership effectiveness and so on.

Gathering Data

There are numerous ways to gather data for assessment. Presented here are brief descriptions for some of the most frequently used methods surveys, rating scales, and qualitative descriptions. *Surveys* are comprehensive and ask for responses to open-ended questions or statements. *Rating scales* are lists of topics, activities, opinions, and the like, to which members assign a rating, such as 5 = good. These are easy to construct, administer, score and can yield valuable information. The results can be compiled by adding the ratings and deriving a total score, derive a mean rating for all items, or compute a mean rating for each item. It could be particularly useful for planning purposes to look at items rated 3 or less by many members, or items mean ratings were 3 or less.

Qualitative Analysis

This too is a specialized field of study encompassing narrative analysis, conversational analysis, fieldwork, ethnography, and case studies. These cannot be easily described, and are too complex to present here. However, if you understand qualitative research methods, such as narrative analysis, you could really derive rich material in analyzing group members' responses to carefully formulated open-ended questions. Both overt and covert meanings can be derived that are good indicators of progress, learning, awareness, and emotionally laden content.

The next two major sections present the importance of the first and closing sessions.

The Critical First Session

The beginning session sets the pattern, tone and expectations for the group and its members, but much of the pattern that emerges is not on a conscious level. The pattern, tone and expectations can be modified as the group progresses or evolves or is changed with the introduction of a new member and/or with the termination of a member, crises, a change in or for the group leader, and so on. Although these are set in the first session, they can be changed but it takes considerable effort to change the pattern.

Facilitating the All-Important First Session

The pattern, tone, and expectations for the group are set in the very first session although much of this is not visible or conscious. This is why it is extremely important for the leader to do all of the following. Organize the first session so that all activities contribute to reduction of ambiguity and uncertainty. Basic tasks for the group leader include calming members' fears, collaboratively set group goals to be consistent with members' goals, review the expectations for behavior and rules, emphasize the limits and expectations for confidentiality and documentation and other ethical concerns, and foster universality and hope all of which can help to begin to build trust and safety.

Calm Fears

Members can be very fearful of the group, especially when the group is their first such experience. Many members will not admit that they are fearful or speak openly about their fears. Indeed, even mentioning the word can arouse resistance. Thus, the group leader has to listen carefully, understand metaphors, and make these fears visible. Additionally, the leader must understand that members use certain words that signal fear in a milder form. Words such as disquiet, dread, apprehensive, and anxious can be substituted for fear, and for some, fear may be too intense to describe what they are experiencing.

   Tip: Group leaders cannot provide enough reassurance to members that they are safe and can trust other members and the leader. Words are not sufficient and leaders who try to answer each fear with logic and rationality run the risk of intensifying the fear and/or arousing other fears.

   Leaders have to become comfortable with allowing members to express their fears, provide minimum reassurance when possible or necessary, respond empathetically to let members know that their fears are understood and acting to reduce the situations that could have the fears realized. It is also important that leaders do not minimize, ignore, overlook, or fail to respond to fears. Members need to feel that the leader is capable of taking care of them, and acknowledging their fears helps with this task.

   Let's examine two common metaphorical statements members may make and questions that may crop up that can be reflective of fears. Also presented are some possible leader responses that try to make the underlying concern or fear more visible.

Situation 1

- **Group member** – "I don't know what this group can do for me."
- **Possible fears** – Fear of not being helped, or of not getting better.
- **Leader acknowledgement** – "You're wondering if you can be helped or to get better. You don't want to be disappointed."

Situation 2

- **Group member** – "Things will get too intense, and I don't like intense situations."
- **Possible fears** – Fear that sessions will get out of control, that they will be hurt or destroyed, or that the leader is not capable of taking care of members.
- **Leader acknowledgment** – "It can be scary when there is a lot of intensity since it is hard to predict what will happen to you. You're wondering if I will be able to manage intense emotions."

In Situation 1 what the leader does not want to do is to provide a list of possible benefits such as, learning coping skills or developing better relationships. Those benefits are probably available in writing and/or were presented verbally, and that's not the real question. It would also be helpful to not say in some form that members will get out of the group what they put into it. That can convey blame and criticism. Recognizing the underlying fear, such as the leader's response in situation 1, is much more helpful.

In Situation 2 the leader may be dealing with several fears including that member's fear of losing control, or of becoming overwhelmed or enmeshed by others' intense feelings. It's too early in the group to focus on a response for this possibility because the therapeutic relationship has not been firmly established. It is better to view these metaphorical statements as a plea for reassurance that the leader is in control and can take care of group members. A response that recognizes this and directly addresses it could be enough for the present.

Review or Establish Group Goals

Group goals and objectives should be reviewed or developed. This is also the time where members can be helped to develop realistic and attainable goals. If goals were developed during orientation these can be reviewed for integration into group goals otherwise pare of first session can be used to survey members about their goals, objectives, and expectations; and to combine and integrate these into realistic, attainable, and agreed-on group goals.

Keep the final goal(s) to bring back to the group for review and evaluation approximately halfway through the life of the group, and at the end of the group. This will help keep members focused on the primary expectations for the group experience.

Expectations for Member's Behavior and Rules

It is helpful to describe what members are expected to do in the group because many of them will come to group not having any notion of how this group experience is different and having some concerns about their expected behavior. They are facing an unknown situation and may be anxious because of the uncertainty and unknown. Thus, it can be very calming to tell members some basic behaviors that can enrich their group experiences. It is probably best to limit these to just a few to discuss verbally, and to give them some guidance. Tell members to practice the following basic behaviors as these are likely to be non-threatening and can be helpful. Ask members to speak of their thoughts, ideas, and feelings as they experience them in the session, to respond directly to other members, ask for what is wanted or needed, take responsibility for their feelings, to make personal statements instead of global or group ones, and to determine the amount and extent of their self-disclosure.

Standards and Rules

The group standards and rules should be verbalized and/or provided in writing to reduce ambiguity and uncertainty. Group leaders will find it helpful to have standards and rules about attendance, missed sessions, arriving on time, and staying the entire session, notification of emergencies and crisis, allowing or not allowing food and drink in the session, policy on coming to sessions under the influence of alcohol and/or illegal drugs, aggressive behavior, contact and /or socializing outside the group guidelines, electronic devices and so on. These can be constructed to meet the group's needs.

Limits for Confidentiality and Requirements for Reporting

Confidentiality is always of concern, but group leaders cannot guarantee that personal disclosures will be kept confidential by all members, however they can request that disclosures in the group be kept confidential including not identifying members in any postings on social media. In addition, there can be legal and/or agency requirements for and these should be revealed to group members prior to the group's beginning. Leaders are also advised to become knowledgeable about the federal HIPPA regulations about reporting and exchange of treatment information, including group members' access to reports and case notes about them and the group.

Group leaders must remain sensitive to the needs and limitations for confidentiality, and specifically address these at the beginning of the group. Group members can be asked to keep personal information disclosed in the group confidential, but are free to disclose the process, materials, and cognitive information.

There is also *privileged communication*, which refers to the extent of privacy in the therapeutic relationship, and the limited right to withhold information from the court. Group leaders need to check the laws in their states, and to know their rights and responsibilities, such as if there is a requirement to respond to a subpoena for records without proper consent, or a court order. Generally, the client has to give consent for release of records, except under narrowly defined circumstances.

The Health Insurance Portability and Accountability Act (HIPAA) of 1996 sets standards for transactions and code sets, unique identifiers, privacy and security for personal health information. The standards delineates what health information may be transmitted, in what form, and to whom. Also covered is the security of this information including how it is kept, stored, transmitted, and/or accessed in electronic form. Information includes any protected health information, such as billing records, insurance reimburse-ments, health care claims, eligibility and coordination of benefits as well as case notes, recordings and other forms of record keeping and documentation. Protection of privacy is the guiding principle.

There are also special confidentiality situations that must be considered under HIPAA; minors, substance abuse, group and family counseling, public offenders, and after a client's death. *Counseling minors* requires par-ental/guardian permission, but the laws and standards for adult con-fidentiality also usually apply to minors. Readers are advised to consult their state laws for applicability to minors in their states, and to be familiar with the Family Educational Rights and Privacy Act of 1974 (FERPA), and with the school board policies of the district when working with children in schools.

There are other ethical concerns such as freedom to exit and group lea-ders should be aware of these and the possible consequences for group members.

Members' Self-disclosure

It can be crucial that an atmosphere receptive to appropriate disclosure be established in the first session. Notice that the term receptive is used, not that disclosure is expected as the first session may be too soon for members to be ready to disclose much of what concerns them. If they are to do so later in the life of the group, what happens during the first session will play major roles in their decision to disclose or not, the level and extent of the disclosure, and in how other members will receive it. Leader actions that facilitate developing an atmosphere receptive to disclosure include non-verbal attending to the speaker, active listening, or empathetic responses, responding directly to each speaker, identification and repair of any empathetic failures that occur. Additional leader actions can include recognizing significant disclosures that are masked, hidden, or expressed as metaphors, blocking verbal attacks, put-downs and sarcastic remarks or responses. rephrasing member comments to highlight feelings and linking members' comments to show commonalities or similarities.

There are also some actions that leaders refrain from doing such as ignoring, overlooking or minimizing a disclosure, suggesting that a disclosure is trivial or meaningless, fail to respond, or to respond directly, push or demand that a member disclose, allowing the leader's personal values to impact or influence their responses to members' disclosures, ignoring empathetic failures, failure to intervene in attacks and the like, and/or indicating verbally or nonverbally that a member is wrong in their expression, thought, feeling or response. Using basic attending skills, having inner resources that are genuine and that promote empathetic responses, and staying in touch with the impact of group experiencing on members are the basics for facilitating disclosure. The first session is extremely important in direct and indirect ways and requires a lot of attention and leader expertise.

Promote Universality and Hope

The tendencies of many group members and some leaders are to stay focused on visible differences and to highlight these. It can be very helpful for some members to have their visible differences acknowledged at some point. Visible differences in gender, age, race/ethnicity, disability, and so on, are very important to these members and they want to know that they are being seen as they are. However, the leader must take care to not rush to highlight these visible differences for the following reasons: all members who are visually different co not want to have those differences high-lighted, focusing on differences can get the misdirected into a prolonged discussion about the impact of these differences and lose the focus for the group, members can imitate the leader and continue to highlight differences instead of searching for similarities, and a difference that is very important to the person can be minimized for example, a member with a visible disability can hear other members minimizing them by saying something like "We all have some disability."

It could be more helpful for the group if the leader would remember the benefits for members perceiving similarities, and to identify and highlight these. Members who have a strong need to have their differences recognized will bring this to the group's attention. The leader then has an opening to address these and other differences that may be in the group.

What may be of more importance for universality are other not so visible similarities, such as past experiences, values, emotional reactions, needs, desires, and fantasies. Any of these, when made visible, can help forge connections at a deeper and more meaningful level.

Strategies for Encouraging Hope

Many group members come to group in a state of hopelessness and despair, and/or having unrealistic expectations for what being in a group can accomplish for them. It is not unusual for members to expect the leader and the group to "fix" whatever they perceive as needing fixing, or to have a mindset that trying to do anything about their situation is futile and hopeless. The group leader can be instrumental in turning these into hope.

It is helpful for the group leader to do the following, and to guide members to do the same.

1 Have a realistic belief about what can be achieved.

- *Examples: Long-term goals can be broken down into short-term goals and progress monitored so that members can begin to recognize progress. Change is possible, but takes time and effort.*

2 Explore with members their beliefs about what can be achieved. This can assist them to be realistic about their expectations and goals.

- *Examples: Focus their thoughts on what they can accomplish that does not involve change on the part of another person.*

3 Concentrate on positive aspects, underused or unrecognized inner resources, personal strengths members have, and possible coping strategies.

- *Example: Identify one or more strengths each member brings to the group, and/or to their situation. Highlight a possible unrealized strength embedded in the self.*

4 Build on, highlight and emphasize whatever is positive in the session.

- *Examples: When members reach out to each other, give support and encouragement and, use that opportunity to comment, praise or explain how that was helpful.*

5 Give members a reason to continue to struggle.

- *Examples: Show your faith in their ability to learn other coping strategies. Empower them to take charge of their growth and development, provide opportunities for them to note (see) how others were successful.*

6 Emphasize positive coping strategies.

- *Examples: Members can share personal coping strategies, and the leader can explore with other members it is possible for them to adapt a particular strategy to meet their personal needs. The leader can propose or suggest strategies that have worked for others.*

Leader Actions – the First Session

Observe interactions among members and with the leader as this provides considerable information about members' characteristic ways of interacting and relating. What members do in the group is reflective of what they do outside the group in other relationships. Some behaviors to note are the following. Don't comment on these or highlight them as it is too soon in the relationship to have the comments received positively.

- Pay attention to members' tendencies to interrupt others and note who interrupts and who is interrupted.
- Story-telling and monopolizing especially when considerable details are presented, and members keep it going with questions.
- Thoughts expressed as feelings.
- Ignoring or minimizing someone's disclosure or feelings.
- Who is excluded, never asked to give an opinion or feeling, and so on.
- Facial expressions when looking at other members
- Eye contact or lack of eye contact when speaking with others. Be sure to remember the cultural component when observing this.
- Projections and possible transference.
- A lack of effort to connect and/or relate.

The pattern for interacting and relating you see in the first session is likely to continue in some way. You can help modify these by teaching more effective ways to interact, communicate and relate, but you need to know members' needs in these areas in order to focus your teaching.

One leader task is to *foster inclusion* of all members. Inclusion is not the same as helping them to feel comfortable in the group, it carries a deeper significance. Don't try to act as a host or hostess, or a social director as this group situation is different. Members who are included feel respected, valued, cared for, and connected at a significant level.

The leader's inner self as genuine, accepting and caring is the major asset for helping members feel included. Behaviors that can help are empathetic listening and responding, soliciting members' feelings and other reactions, patience with resistance and defensiveness and not try to battle them into agreement or submission, and by providing encouragement and support.

The group's pattern for interacting, disclosure, relating and acceptance is set in the first session, but it is difficult to see except in retrospect. There can be adaptations, adjustments, and modifications for the pattern, but the essential nature will remain throughout the group. The actual acts will change, but not the underlying pattern.

The pattern, tone, and expectations are greatly influenced by what the leader does and says. For example, if the leader encourages members to ask questions, then much of the interaction and verbalization will be in the form of questions, not just about the cognitive material, but also when members are trying to relate to each other. Leaders have to understand that their unconscious and nonconscious behavior and attitudes are being observed and responded to more than their conscious ones. Members try to give leaders what they think the leader wants, although none of this is spoken. Other examples can include the following:

- If a leader fails to recognize emotional intensity, members can refrain from verbalizing deep and intense feelings.
- If a leader is not alert to metaphors, member can feel the leader does not, or cannot understand.
- When the leader fails to make an empathetic response, members can feel devalued, minimized, or even shamed.
- If a leader assumes that they are the expert, members will be reluctant to contribute their knowledge and wisdom.

The following outline lists the leader's tasks to reduce ambiguity and uncertainty:

- Formulate specific goal(s) and objectives to include members' goals. This is a collaborative task.
- Develop a short list of rules and distribute these in writing.
- Lead a discussion on confidentiality, the requirements for reporting, and the limits imposed on the leader.
- Introductions for members and the leader.
- Initiate a discussion about expectations for participation, self-disclosure and the like.
- Restrict questioning by the leader, and from the members. Limit questions from members to factual information unless there is something urgent and important brought to the group.
- Openly acknowledge that the group can seem ambiguous, and that new situations arouse uncertainty.
- Allow members to express their anxiety and make empathetic responses.
- Summary for the session.

The Importance of Planned Group Closure

Closure is the term used, instead of termination, as it denotes a process where termination tends to denote an end. It can be important for the group leader to have a deep understanding of the need for a process to end the group rather than abruptly ending, or worse, no definitive ending of the group. Leaders should make closure a part of the planning process and use the expected member behavior, feelings and attitudes described in stage 4 as a guide for what to expect. The leader's own experiences with loss, saying goodbye, and unfinished business can have an unconscious impact on the extent to which they approach planned closure for groups.

The benefits or value of planned closure include the following:

- A boundary is established, agreed to, and understood by all members at both the cognitive and affective levels.
- Time is allocated for the completion of unfinished business.

- Members are taught a process for saying goodbye.
- Focus is on essentials of the experience and the relationships
- The leader demonstrates how to work through loss and grief.
- Validation and legitimization of sadness.

The Time Boundary

Many types of groups have a specific *time frame* for existence, but others may not have a specific time for ending. A process for individual termination and premature termination are described in a separate section. This section focuses on closure for time bound or time limited groups where all members are terminating.

Even when there is a specific time frame for the group, some members may carry an incomplete understanding on a nonconscious level that the group will end. This can be especially troublesome for members who are profiting from the experience, value the learning and relationships established, and who don't want the good feelings of stage 3 to disappear. These are the members who will deny to themselves that the group is ending. There can be other members who did not consciously realize the value and importance of the group for them until the very end, and they too can be oblivious to the ending of the group.

It can be helpful for group leaders to begin the closure process about halfway through the duration for the group by stating how many sessions are left. It isn't necessary to do this every remaining session but should be done often enough so that members don't lose sight or awareness of it. The issues to be addressed for closure include decreasing unfinished business, working through grief and loss, reflection on gain and progress, and expression of feelings about the experience.

Unfinished Business

Almost everyone has some unfinished business where they did not say or do some things, the relationship stopped or ended, and they are left with regrets, yearnings or wishes about the person or the relationship. The group is an opportunity to prevent this from happening once again, to demonstrate the value of completing and communicating feelings and thoughts to each other, and to experience the feelings of a satisfactory ending to relationships.

Closure is the time where members can say those things they want the other person to know, usually positive. What many people regret is that they did not tell someone that they were liked, appreciated, respected, admired for a trait or action, and so on. While there can be unfinished business about negative or uncomplimentary things, most of these would satisfy a revenge need, such as a pay-back for real or imagined offenses. These too can carry regrets, but not as much as failure to say positive things do.

A Process for Saying Goodbye

These are reasons for members to stay in touch with the real impending closure of the group, to use a process for saying goodbye that includes speaking their thoughts, feelings, and so on, in the group. That way they will not be left with much or any unfinished business relative to the group. Members may have to be taught how to phrase comments they think have the potential for negative reception. Both leaders and members may need to say things that are uncomplimentary, such as telling someone that they have a habit of interrupting others. The basic guidelines for phrasing what may be a negative comment are as follows.

- Doing so to help the other person become aware of the impact of the particular behavior on oneself-not on others.
- Having motives for telling this that do not include revenge or superiority.
- Phrasing it carefully with sensitivity to the impact the words have on the received.
- Limiting it to a particular action, behavior, or situation.
- Focusing on something that can be changed not something that is fixed.
- Do not use words such as; always, never, good, bad, right, or wrong.

It is possible to tell someone how you feel about them, or the behavior that may be negative, without blaming or criticizing. Members can be made aware that this group is an opportunity to leave a relationship or experience without carrying unfinished business.

Tip: One strategy leaders can use to help members understand and accept the importance of satisfactory closure is to ask members how do they usually say goodbye. Ask them to reflect on the experiences and relationships in their past, and how they ended them.

It will be unusual to not have several members who do not say good-bye at all, or who find ways to avoid saying it. They just leave, don't show up or even call on the last day, substitute a social or other activity so that is becomes too busy to say good-bye or make sure they are a part of a group saying goodbye. It is also unusual to find that most members are satisfied with how they have said goodbye.

If you don't take the time to say goodbye, you can be left with residual feelings of regret. Yes, it can be painful and difficult to look at someone, know that you will never or are unlikely to ever see them again, feel sad about the loss of the connection, and have the courage to tell that person how much you have appreciated them and valued the relationship, and the sense of loss you are experiencing at saying goodbye.

Tip: Tell group members that it is important to say goodbye in some way, and explore with them the possible means of doing so. It is important to do this as saying goodbye is a necessary part of letting go.

Focusing on Essentials

Having to say goodbye and let go can assist members in focusing on the essentials of the experience and of the relationship with each member and the leader. It is not sufficient to just focus on the group as a whole, it is also necessary to reflect on experiences and responses to each individual member, and with the leader. Members may want to reflect on questions such as the following:

- What actions, attitudes, responses and so on, were helpful during group sessions?
- Who did I have strong reactions to (both positive and negative) and what produced these?
- How did my perceptions, reactions, and the like of group members and/or the leader change over the course of the group?
- What do I want to make sure is said before the group ends?
- What do I value about the group, the members and the leader?
- What am I taking away as a result of this group experience?

Working through Grief and Loss

It would be unusual to have a group where members had not experienced grief and loss in their lives. Indeed, some members will be experiencing these as a result of their illness or condition, giving the leader a great opportunity to demonstrate a process for working through them. In addition, closure can also bring up unresolved grief and loss, and generate its own sense of grief and loss around the ending of the group. When grief becomes prolonged, intense, or complicated, the normal grief behaviors are increased, and other troubling behaviors and attitudes added. This state requires specialized treatment, and it is mentioned here because group leaders may encounter this with some unresolved grief issues members may have.

Leaders can adapt the following process for demonstrating how to work through grief and loss:

1   Acceptance of the end or loss.
2   Express feelings about loss.
3   Deal with the memories.
4   Readjust to changes.
5   Build new relationships.

Leader task: One leader task is to validate the sadness experienced by members around closure.
Validation of sadness means that:

- Expressions of loss and sadness are recognized even when expressed as metaphors.

- Empathetic responses are made.
- Other group members are invited to give their reactions to the expression of sadness.
- The validity of the ending of the group is affirmed.
- Members are asked for suggestions about a satisfactory ending for each of them.

Unanticipated and Difficult Closures – Premature Termination

It is much easier to plan closure for the group as a whole than it is for an individual member, such as what occurs in support groups, where members can terminate at any time. There are other situations that can also present difficult closure; the death of a member, relapse or another illness, moving away, military service, a member just decides to leave or stop attending without notice, family crises that affect attendance, the breakup of a romantic relationship established between two group members, reduced income, and so-on. What all or most of these situations have in common, is that in advance they tend to be unexpected. This is why leaders should plan in advance for possible premature termination, as it has a definite impact on the group and on the members.

Members can be encouraged to give notification in advance when they intend to terminate especially before the group is supposed to end. That can mean that members who desire or intend to leave the group are expected to notify the leader as far in advance as possible. This notification can give the leader an opportunity to prepare that member and the group for the departure. Leaders can assist the member in announcing the intent to the group, deciding on how much information should be communicated about the reason or circumstances for leaving, facilitate members saying goodbye, and empathetically responding to the loss of that member.

Much more difficult to handle will be the unexpected circumstance, such as death or no information about why the member leaves. These unexpected terminations can arouse deep feelings about abandonment, personal failings, and other such emotions that arise from the various members' family of origin and other past experiences. It is not unusual for some members to feel that they did something to "cause" that member to leave. Adding to the complexity is that some members experience these emotions, but do not openly verbalize them. Leaders may not be aware of the possibility of these emotions and do not do anything that could help these members work through them.

Care should be taken to not minimize or overlook the impact the unexpected leaving can have on members. This is a case where something urgent and important occurs for the group, and that takes priority over whatever was planned. This is where leaders can be most helpful in leading members to become aware of and work through their feelings about the particular member, the unexpected termination, and residual feelings about other unsatisfactory terminations they may have experienced.

Leaders should also stay in touch with what they are feeling and use this inner experiencing as a way to help group members express what they may be feeling. It is not appropriate for leaders to work on their issues that cause the feelings, but it is appropriate for them to report their feelings to the group. This permits the leader to teach members how to address losses from the past, in the present, and for the future.

Closure is as important and difficult as is the successful beginning of the group and needs careful attention and consideration by the leader. This is another instance where the extent of the leader's personal development can be helpful in providing inner guidance about what to say and do to assist group members, and leaders are encouraged to think, reflect, and plan for closure of all types.

References

AGPA & IBCGP. (2002). *Guidelines for Ethics in Group Psychotherapy*. New York: American Group Psychotherapy Association & International Board of Certified Group Psychotherapists.

Brown, N. (2003). *Psychoeducational Groups* (2nd edition). New York: Routledge.

Burlingame, G., Cox, J., Davis, R., Layne, C., & Gleave, R. (2011). The group selection questionnaire: Further refinements in group member selection. *Group Dynamics: Theory, Research, and Practice*, 15(1), 60–74.

Gans, J. S. & Alonso, A. (1998). Difficult patients: Their construction in group therapy. *International Journal of Group Psychotherapy*, 48(3), 311–326.

Kalodner, C. R., & Coughlin, J. W. (2004). Psychoeducational and counseling groups to prevent and treat eating disorders and disturbances. In J. L. DeLucia-Waack, C. R. Kalodner, & M. Riva (Eds.), *Handbook of Group Counseling and Psychotherapy*, pp 481–496. Thousand Oaks, CA: Sage Publications.

MacNair-Semands, R. R., & Lese, K. P. (2000). Interpersonal problems and the perception of therapeutic factors in group therapy. *Small Group Research*, 31, 158–174.

5 Group Sessions and Members

Developmental Group Stages

Tuckman (1965) was among the first to propose and document developmental sequences for groups, and this later became known as group stages. These stages are not separate, distinct, or clear-cut, but almost all types of groups seem to move through some sequence of development.

Proposed here is a model that incorporates much of what is presented in the literature and adds major leader tasks, and major member concerns for each stage. The discussion about each stage also includes some hidden and/or unexpressed member concerns that may be present. There are four stages in the model: meaning and purpose, challenges, unfolding and becoming, and closure (Brown, 2009).

Stage 1: The Beginning Stage

Members will be seeking meaning and purpose for their being in the group and will have varying degrees of concerns. The major member concerns are safety, inclusion, personal gains, and symptom relief. *Safety* concerns can be mild or extensive depending on the member's past experiences. Basically, they are concerned and apprehensive about being shamed or humiliated by the leader or by other members. They can fear appearing stupid or incompetent where others will ridicule, embarrass, or devalue them in some way, and this would be painful to endure. Members will also have concerns about being *included* in the group as they do not yet know what the overt and covert norms will be. Everyone carries secrets about their self, and some of these can be shame producing, which arouses fear of being discovered, revealed, or disclosed. If the feared action was to occur, the overriding concern is about being too flawed to be acceptable and thus, will be excluded.

Every member has some level of concern about what they can *gain from being in the group*. Even involuntary members who may be extremely resistant want to know what's in it for them. If members cannot see any positive benefits or outcomes for participation, they do not commit to the

DOI: 10.4324/9781003329787-5

group, their level of investment and involvement is minimal at best, and their anxiety levels remain high. *Symptom relief* is sought by some members, and this need or wish can be realistic or unrealistic. That is, the symptoms may not be addressed by this group, it may not be possible to provide the desired relief, or the focus may be on the wrong symptoms.

The *Beginning* stage could be called the sorting through and connecting process and there is no set time for when it ends. Members are generally strangers to each other, confused and frustrated with the ambiguity and the unknown about the group, fearful of being rejected or excluded, and concerned that their flaws, shameful secrets, and desires will become visible to all. In addition, they may be carrying considerable stress over their illness, condition and/or other life situation, and have intense uncomfortable emotions they are trying to manage. Members can have questions about the efficacy of group for their personal need, and mistrust and/or fear about the competency and ability of the leader to take care of them. Most often, none of this is directly expressed, but emerges through metaphors. In addition to sorting through all these, formulating goals, and deciding how much of the real self can be shown in the group, members are also trying to make connections to other members and to the leader. This too takes place in a variety of ways. What can be important for all leaders to try to do is to support the attempts to make connections by focusing on significant, but not visible, commonalities. It's easy to spot commonalities such as age, gender, and race/ethnicity much of the time, and revealed commonalities such as education, marital status, geographic location, careers or jobs, hobbies, and recreational pursuits. These are surface similarities that probably do not help members become connected at meaningful levels. Those connections seem to be forged around shared intense experiences that continue to carry meaning for the members, deeply held values and other principles that guide their lives, similar emotions around a common event that occurs in the group, and similar self-perceptions around similar issues or concerns. The visible and revealed similarities are those that emerge in social situations, tend to be non-threatening to the person(s) involved, and don't have intense emotions associated with them. These could be called benign similarities whereas meaningful connections are at a deeper level. Leaders will probably not be able to help members connect at a very deep and meaningful level, especially in the beginning stage, but can help this occur by linking the more meaningful similarities whenever they appear, even in the first session, and by having this as a priority for their work with the group. It is always helpful to keep in mind that members become cohesive around similarities and fail to do so when differences are paramount.

Vignette

This is the third meeting for the group composed of 8 college students aged 18–22. The group was required for all students who violated the college's policy on alcohol use. The first two meetings focused on introductions, goal setting and getting acquainted. This session started quietly with members reporting on their weekly activities. However, about 15 minutes into the 2 hour session, members began to ramble and talk about topics that did not appear to be group related. The topics included difficulty in finding a parking space, the Survivor television show, an unfair boss at work, and nosey siblings. The leader let the rambling proceed for a few minutes.

Reflection/discussion: How are the members' basic concerns for stage 1 reflected in this group session?

Member Behaviors

Member behaviors in stage 1 are fueled by their anxiety and fear, and the pattern for their relating to each other and to the leader is largely determined by their family of origin experiences, past experiences, and unfinished business and/or unresolved issues from these. Expected member feelings can include confusion, fear or dread, irritation or anger, resentment, defiance, and shame. Members are confused about the ambiguity that surrounds the unknown experience of this group, they can fear or dread exclusion or rejection by other members and by the leader, there can be irritation or anger about their conditions that brought them to the group and/or at other external people and situations, resentment at being as or where they are, defiant of authority as located in the leader or of the forces that sent them to the group, and shame about many aspects of self.

Expected member behaviors in stage 1 include the following.

- Expressions of discontent that are indirect and disguised.
- Considerable questioning where given answers do not appear to be satisfactory and continue to be repeated in different ways.
- Expressions of frustration and anger at external events, people and the like.
- Talking only to the leader, and seldom if ever to each other.
- Saying and doing things so as to be perceived as nice and cooperative.
- Frequently saying "I don't understand".

Tip: Leaders' tasks are to contain and manage anxiety both personal and that of members, to reduce ambiguity surrounding the group process, to forge a therapeutic relationship with members, to help set group goals and group norms, and to begin establishing trust and safety in the group. The members are still searching for purpose and safety, and are concerned about confidentiality and if they can be helped. There is considerable unspoken anxiety about these topics, and the verbalized topics are metaphors.

The major *tasks for the leader* focus on setting a group atmosphere where members can feel safe, promoting inclusion, and reducing fears and anxiety.

Basic and fundamental leader actions to accomplish these tasks include providing information about the leader's qualifications, the intended purpose for the group, guiding members to set reasonable rules and regulations for the group, identifying possible concerns and expectations about confidentiality, soliciting input from all members, engaging in collaborative goals setting, and designing activities to help members begin to become acquainted. It is also helpful to have group members discuss any fears or apprehensions they have about the group and their participation.

Stage 2: Dissatisfaction, Conflict, and Challenges

Let's return to the group described for the first stage for a different session later in the group.

Vignette

It is now a later session, and the members can only be described as very quiet and withdrawn. The leader wonders what happened since the previous session seemed to go very well with all members participating, interactions among members increased, some significant self-disclosures were made, and members said they were pleased with their progress. However, this session is a complete reversal of the previous one.

The group began in silence, and no one spoke unless addressed directly by the leader, and then the speaker was very terse without volunteering any additional information. The leader asked what was happening to change the mood from the previous session, but no one responded. The leader then produced an exercise to try to overcome the stuck feeling, members completed it, but there was no energy around it, and it did not seem to produce any insight or learning. The session ended as it began, with silence.

The next session was even more different. Members were cranky and irritable, challenging and arguing with each other over almost everything that was said. The leader tried to intervene but was ignored. Finally, one member said angrily and loudly that he was bored, tired of the group, and didn't feel he as being helped. Some other members said that they felt the same way, and that the group wasn't going anywhere.

Expected Member Behaviors

There are not clear demarcations between stages so it can be difficult at times to determine which stage is most prevalent for a group. Since the leader's tasks and interventions can be different, it can be important to be able to identify when the group seems to be in stage 2 as this is the most uncomfortable of the stages for the leader and for group members. Some identifiers include the following member behaviors.

- Challenges to the leader's competence and/or authority.
- Expressions of discontent about the course or progress of the group.
- An emphasis on differences among group members.

- Expressions of irritation to each other and/or to the leader.
- More open expressions of negative responses to each other.
- Efforts to exert power and control.
- More visible projections and transference.
- Few empathetic or understanding responses by group members.
- Open conflict with the leader and/or other members.

This stage is marked by dissent and conflict, some of which is passive or disguised, and some may be openly expressed. How the group leader manages their reactions and feelings about conflict will mainly determine how group members manage conflict in the group or if they will avoid, ignore or minimize. Group members will take their cues about conflict from observing the group leader.

The very idea of conflict is very disturbing to many group leaders and members. To some, it is so threatening that they work hard to keep it from appearing in the group, failing to realize or accept that conflict does not have to be destructive, it can be managed in a way that it accomplishes all of the following.

- Increases understanding of self and others.
- Makes visible unconscious projections and transference.
- Allows uncomfortable feelings to be expressed and explored as catharsis and interpersonal learning.
- Teaches how to contain and manage one's personal feelings, such as anger and hurt.
- Shows how to let go of grudges and resentments.
- Can strengthen relationships.
- Highlights closely held perceptions of authority and sibling relationships.

Thus, leaders should strive to become more comfortable with some level of conflict, accept and understand its importance for group progress, and learn how to make constructive use of it. Members will catch the leader's attitude and feelings about conflict, put their own spin on it, and act on it in some way.

Tip: How can a leader know that conflict is being resisted by group members? Some clues can be an insistence on describing the group as cohesive in the beginning stage, making comments about how well they are getting along, a quick and unquestioning acceptance of whatever the leader and other members propose, non-verbal behavior that communicates a desire for flight and/or considerable discomfort in the group, provocative or teasing comments, sarcasm, quick soothing and reassuring responses when a member or the leader seems annoyed, and a minimizing of differences among members and with the leader.

During this stage is also the time when group members begin to assert their individuality, experiment with new or different behaviors, connect with each other through their commonalties, and start to become less reliant on the leader. Disagreements and other forms of conflict emerge, and how these are managed is a strong determiner of whether or not the cooperative and productiveness of stage 3 is achieved.

The *leader's major tasks* for stage 2 are to recognize attacks and challenges, manage their and members' personal anxiety and defensiveness, block attacks on members by other members, to not engage in attacks on members either directly or indirectly, to teach conflict resolution skills, reframe disagreements and other such remarks, and to highlight empathic failures and repair them.

Stage 3: Cohesion

Vignette

During a later session for the same group, the leader observes members responding directly with each other, making reflective or empathic responses, engaging in significant self-disclosures, and generally working well together. It is a very different group from when it began, and as it was just a couple of sessions ago.

The group feels wonderful, valued and productive at this stage. However, the leader must stay aware that members can become reluctant to do or say anything that has the potential to destroy this harmony and pleasant feeling, so negative responses and feelings can be suppressed. This is also the stage where cliques can form and exert a felt negative impact. Cliques will be impossible to prevent as members will get to know each other and forge meaningful connections. Then too, if the members are together in a setting, such as a hospital or rehabilitation center, they can or will have considerable interactions outside the group, and this can also facilitate the emergence of cliques. Members not in the clique can feel excluded, that secrets are being shared outside the group, and that clique members have a certain bond that encourages an "us against them" attitude.

Tip: The most group leaders can do to nullify these possible negative effects of a clique is to emphasize that group matters are not to be discussed outside the group, even among group members. Leaders will not be able to enforce this, but the awareness of what behavior is expected can help prevent some of this. Other than emphasizing this, there is not much else available to group leaders. They can discuss the negative effects of cliques, or ask that topics discussed outside the group be brought back to the group, but that cannot be enforced. Cliques promote secrecy and mistrust. Most group members will want to avoid these.

Expected Member Behaviors

Expected member behaviors in stage 3 include expressing immediate feelings and reactions directly to other members and to the leader, making personal statements such as I or me, acknowledging and accepting similarities, engaging in catharsis that includes interpersonal learning, responding empathetically and giving and receiving constructive feedback. Attitudes can include considerably less defensive behavior and resistance, increased awareness of self and others, and a sense of the group as a safe place to let the real self appear.

Tip: Leader's main tasks at this stage are to stay out of the way so that members can work; identify group resistance; make group process commentary to help members become more aware of what they are collectively doing; encourage and support members' self-exploration; highlight members' growth, development and progress; and to use the therapeutic factors that emerge.

Major leader tasks during the stage are few since members come prepared to work and engage in effective member behaviors. This is the stage where group process commentary is most effective as members are more open to reflecting on the commentary, and do not immediately reject it unexamined. Leaders have to be careful to not push members too much, to let them work through disagreements and clashes, refrain from intervening too quickly, and to give members more leeway in self-examination and self-exploration. Another possible threat to the group's progress can be members' unwillingness to bring up negative responses and reactions among group members. Leaders can ask if members are suppressing these as a way to remind them that progress can be made when members can be genuine.

Stage 3 is the stage where both task and relationship factors combine to foster collaborative task accomplishment. Individual members are helped to achieve their personal goals through the combined resources of the group as a whole, and other members. Members' primary concerns are harmony, providing constructive and helpful interpersonal feedback, increasing awareness of self and of others, and personal growth in understanding or skills, and so on.

The major group *leader task* for this stage of development is to stay out of the way and let the members work, and to help guide members to work through rather than suppressing even minor conflicts. There can be a reluctance among members to do or say anything that has the potential for discord. The transition to the ending or termination stage when group members' behavior begins to be more reflective of their behavior in stages 1 and 2, and the harmony and warmth that characterize stage 3 begins to drift away.

Stage 4: Ending or Termination

Vignette

Although the leader has continually reminded members that the group is scheduled to end, members have ignored this ending for several sessions. It is now the next to last session, and members are still refusing to directly consider the group's ending.

Members begin topics and then drop them, they interrupt each other, many empathic failures occur, and the general mood is one of irritability and somberness.

Members can have mixed feelings about ending the group. There can be a sense of relief that they survived the experience, pleasure at realizing the growth and development they made, regret for missed opportunities, sadness for loss of meaningful connections made as a result of the group experience, panic at the thought that the group will end before they are ready or have completed their work, and excitement or despair about their futures. Each member will have different feelings. The leader's task is to prepare members for closure of this experience in a way that leaves them with few or no regrets, or a sense of unfinished business.

It is essential that leaders plan for termination and not just have the group stop. Members need to be prepared for the ending in sufficient time to internalize it and make their personal adjustments, and to be shown how to effectively end experiences and relationships. Leaders will find that few people know how to do this, or who practice this. Thus, the ending of the group can be an opportunity for further learning for members.

The final stage of the group is also where existential issues can emerge, or re-emerge, and become acute, although this is likely to happen in disguised ways. Existential issues of death, loneliness, alienation and the human conditions of pain and suffering can be a significant part of members' termination fears and process. Their physical and/or mental conditions that brought them to group are still of concern, and may not have improved, or may have even worsened. They can begin to retreat from reaching out to others back to self-absorption. The loss of group support and encouragement is major and significant and should not be minimized, although some members will do this as a way to cope with loss and grief.

Leaders can expect the group to go through some variation of the grieving process: shock and numbness, denial, anger, attempts to make the group continue, and acceptance and accommodation. This is a process that may not be fully accomplished for some members, but any progress is better than none. The need for a satisfactory group termination is crucial, and leaders should begin the process approximately halfway through the life of the group. A process for termination is described in Chapter 4 If the group is open-ended, members should be encouraged to notify the leader several sessions before they intend to terminate. This will allow the leader to guide that member, and the members that remain in the group, through the process.

Tip: The termination stage can see members' behavior regress to stage 1 behavior in some ways. Expected member behaviors can include denial that the group is ending, increased crankiness, suppression of feelings, and withdrawal, minimizing the value of the group, the leader, or what has been gained, panic at the thought of the loss of support provided by the group. In addition, some or all of these can appear: reemergence of dependency on the leader, depression and/or despair about "getting better", confusion about the ambiguity and ambivalent feelings about termination and feelings of abandonment.

Interventions include highlighting members' progress and accomplishments, illustrating how goals were met, teaching members satisfactory closure for the group, and for relationships, providing encouragement, support, and faith in members' abilities to continue to grow and develop and modeling strategies for coping with loss and grief.

It is important that closure not be minimized, truncated, or ignored. Save a social event for after the session, and do not let such activities substitute for closure. Saying goodbye is as important as saying hello.

Stage 4 is the final stage of ending the group experience. Members' concerns and initial feelings seem to re-emerge, some members can panic about the ending because there is so much that seems unfinished, the potential loss of meaningful relationships and support, and other separation issues bubble up and affect the group. It is very important to prepare members for the group's ending, and leaders should plan in advance how this will be handled.

Some members will openly admit to feelings of sadness about the ending of the group and the impact of the loss on them, but many will suppress their feelings or even deny having them. Leaders can find it difficult to get members to express any sadness, and this should be accepted, and members not pushed to voice sadness. Some members will devalue what they did get from the group, the members and/or the leader, some will make depreciating comments, and/or say that it wasn't enough or what was wanted. Members can also resist ending the group by planning a social event as the last session, refusing to discuss ending or deny that they have feelings about the group's ending, initiating conflict in the hope that the leader will not let the group end without resolution of it, and by even asking the leader to meet for additional sessions or voting to continue the group. The leader must resist being seduced into not honoring the contract that was set in the beginning about the number of sessions.

A major way by which members resist ending the group is by bringing up new material to demonstrate that the group is needed to help members work on these important things such as, learn more skills, or address deep issues. The leader is faced with the inner personal need or desire to not leave the member unfulfilled or dangling, to assist in learning or exploration of new material on the one hand, but also the need to honor the contract and end the group. It can be of little help to understand that the presentation of new material is a delaying tactic. Leaders will be very conflicted at this point. However, the responsible response is to acknowledge the seriousness and importance of the new material, the sadness and dismay at not having sufficient time to work on it, but to continue to end the group. Leaders should also check-in with the member who surfaced the new material to ensure that they are able to handle it.

It can be helpful to have two evaluative actions as a part of closure, written and/or oral. A written evaluation is a survey of the group components such as goals, activities, and the leader, and an oral evaluation can be a method of reflection, summarization, appreciation and/or regrets.

Ending a group can be emotionally intense at times, but group leaders should not seek to avoid this intensity as it can be a valuable learning experience for some members to learn how to say good-bye in a more satisfying way so that there is minimal or no unfinished business.

Ethics and Professional Standards

Ethics and professional standards are the rules of conduct governing the members of a professional organization that define the system of moral principles and define good or right behavior. Legal concerns refer to the federal, state, and local laws that apply to profession. All mental health professionals have ethical standards, and members in that profession are expected to know these and to abide by them as these standards guide the professional counselor, and protect clients. Professionals are also expected to be familiar with the federal, state, and local laws that relate to their practice and professional performance. Little is provided in the literature that focuses on ethics for and about groups that is different from other modalities with the exceptions of the ethical guidelines provided by the American Group Psychotherapy Association and the International Board of Certified Group Psychotherapists (AGPA & IBCGP, 2002) and the training manual Ethics in Group Psychotherapy (MacNair-Semands, 2015). Presented here are the general categories for ethics and professional standards for group leaders that include professional preparation and competence, relationship standards, privacy and confidentiality to include HIPPA, technology and documentation, professional boundaries and duties to warn and protect.

Professional Preparation

Professional preparation requires successful completion of prescribed coursework in a formal academic program, practica, and supervised internship and residency programs at a minimum. Specialties require coursework and supervised practice beyond the minimum. It is ethically responsible to practice within the scope of competence, which is based on knowledge, skills, supervised practice, and the work context. *Competency* specifies areas for practice as emotional competence, competence with diverse populations, and conscientious further education. Emotional competence refers to the therapist's emotional and psychological state. Personal problems, compassion fatigue, and burnout can lead to impaired clinical judgment, disrespecting clients, neglecting symptoms, and other such reduction of competence. Competence with diverse populations is self-explanatory but needs emphasizing as the importance of cultural and diversity factors for therapeutic effectiveness continue to be highlighted in the research. *Impairment* is anything, such as a condition or disease, that interferes with the group leader's ability to provide professional and responsible treatment. An impaired group leader puts members and the group at risk of being harmed, and of failing to receive proper care and treatment. There are other conditions and diseases that lead to impaired cognitive functioning where the results would also be detrimental to the group.

The group leader has an ethical responsibility to monitor their physical, mental, and emotional condition and actions for signs of impairment, and to take action to address these, including self-reporting to the supervisor or licensing board. Failure to do so can lead to being less effective as a group leader or even doing harmful things, and failing to take needed actions that would benefit group members. Do no harm sounds simple but may be more difficult to carry out. Lilenfeld's (2007) study provides a list of potentially harmful treatments. Group leaders are unlikely to intentionally harm group members, but there is a vast territory for unintentional harm.

Relationship Standards

Relationship standards for group therapy includes attending to informed consent and freedom to exit. *Informed consent* refers to providing group members with sufficient information that they are able to evaluate the personal risks and benefits for the proposed group. Group members have a right to know this information in advance of participation. Basic information needed for informed consent includes the following:

1 Purpose and goals for the group
2 Techniques to be used
3 General procedures
4 Potential risks and gains for participation
5 The group leader's credentials
6 Screening procedures when these are used
7 Consent forms and treatment plans.

Freedom to exit gives members the right to leave the group at any time. It is an assurance that they will not be forced to remain in the group against their will. However, there are penalties for some group members that can make leaving the group not a viable choice such as when members are court mandated to attend the group. Group leaders need to understand and practice freedom to exit, to not try to force members to remain in the group, and to let it be the member's decision to remain or to leave.

Privacy and Confidentiality

Privacy and confidentiality standards include documentation and reporting responsibilities for the group leader as well as confidentiality, HIPPA regulations privileged communications and privacy. *Confidentiality* is always of concern, even in highly information dissemination non–clinical groups. Leaders cannot guarantee that personal disclosures will be kept confidential by all members, but can request this, and speak of the leader's intentions. In addition, there can be legal requirements for reporting that the leader must obey, and these should be revealed to group members prior to the group's beginning. There can be state and local laws that also affect confidentiality, as well as agency or institutional policies. Leaders should be very aware of all requirements, limitations and the like, that affect confidentiality.

Group leaders must remain sensitive to the needs and limitations for confidentiality, and specifically address these at the beginning of the group. Group members can be asked to keep personal information disclosed in the group confidential, but are free to disclose the process, materials, and cognitive information.

Privileged communication refers to the extent of privacy in the therapeutic relationship, and the limited right to withhold information from the court. Attorneys and clergy have privileged communication rights with their clients in every state. Group leaders need to check the laws in their states, and to know their rights and responsibilities, such as if there is a requirement to respond to a subpoena for records without proper consent, or a court order. Generally, the client has to give consent for release of records, except under narrowly defined circumstances.

The Health Insurance Portability and Accountability Act (HIPAA) of 1996 sets standards for transactions and code sets, unique identifiers, *privacy* and security for personal health information. The standards delineate what health information may be transmitted, in what form, and to whom. Also covered is the security of this information including how it is kept, stored, transmitted, and/or accessed in electronic form. Information includes any protected health information, such as billing records, insurance reimbursements, health care claims, eligibility and coordination of benefits as well as case notes, recordings and other forms of record keeping and documentation. Group leaders are also advised to become knowledgeable about the federal HIPPA regulations about reporting and exchange of treatment information, including group members' access to reports and case notes about them and the group. These regulations describe what information can be shared with others, under what conditions, and need for consent; how the information can be conveyed; and other restrictions and limitations.

There are also special confidentiality situations that must be considered under HIPAA; minors, substance abuse, group and family counseling, public offenders, and after a client's death. *Counseling minors* requires parental/guardian permission, but the laws and standards for adult confidentiality also usually apply to minors. Readers are advised to consult their state laws for applicability to minors in their states, and to be familiar with the Family Educational Rights and Privacy Act of 1974 (FERPA), and with the school board policies of the district when working with children in schools. Confidentiality for *deceased clients* is still protected under many circumstances, and the ACA code recognizes that there may be situations where confidentiality cannot be maintained. The inability to maintain confidentiality for deceased clients may be required by law, the agency's policy, and/or state stature that permits access by the administrator or executor of the estate. Documentation provides evidence of what was done, and group members' progress. Bennett et al. (2006) propose adequate documentation as a means to help reduce risk and as a basic in ethical practice. Examples of documentation include case notes, recordings, mandated and optional reports to others. Standards and expectations for documentation are found in state laws and state regulation boards, professional organizations' standards, and by insurers. Group leaders should know the various federal, state, and institutional requirements for record keeping, including the content and laws governing privileged communications.

Technology and Documentation

Technology and documentation can also present ethical dilemmas. The use of technology for generating and storing case notes, personal notes, session recordings, reports, and all forms of documentation is increasing at a phenomenal rate. Medical records are computerized, and other medical and insurance professionals can have access to the electronically stored records. These can be instances when the court can also obtain these records, and it is only the viability of the computer system's security measures that prevent unauthorized people from access.

Group leaders should remain highly aware of the sensitivity of information in documents, and of the possibility of unauthorized access to them as well as the client's legal rights for access and for privacy. These are important concerns that should guide your record keeping, report generation, and how this information is presented and framed.

Professional Boundaries

Professional boundaries refer to dual relationships including sexual concerns and dual roles. *Dual relationships* are to be avoided where possible and, if avoidance is not possible, care must be taken by the leader to ensure that harm to the client does not result from the dual relationship. The American Psychological Association's 2006 ethics report noted that 36 percent of the dual relationship cases opened were for non-sexual violations, and 64 percent for sexual misconduct with an adult or a minor, and sexual harassment. Other areas of sexual misconduct that merit attention by group leaders are sexual exploitation, and after therapy sexual involvement. *Sexual concerns* include sexual harassment, sexually provocative behavior remarks and the like, seduction, the act of sex with a client, and handling of sexual overtures by clients. In all cases, the group leader should remain aware of the vulnerability of the client, the need for safety and trust for the relationship, the ethical and legal standards and requirements, and their own professional responsibilities. Most if not all ethical standards about sex with a client directly and forcibly state that sex with a client is unethical. There are also dual relationships where the leader and a member(s) have a significant relationship outside the group that is non-sexual such as need not be an intimate one, such as attending parties, weddings and the like; work relationships with regular, evaluative and/or supervisory requirements; educational such as teacher and student, and so on, but the defining role is one that could negatively affect either the leader or member, or both. It is recommended that group leaders consult with supervisors, personal therapists, or colleagues when issues and/or concerns about dual relationships emerge.

It is extremely important for group leaders to maintain their professional boundaries, and to manage and contain their sexual feelings. These feelings can emerge during therapy and/or group sessions and should be dealt with using the assistance of the supervisor and/or personal therapist.

Duties to Warn and Protect

Duties to report, warn, and protect can be both ethical and legal for certain circumstances and conditions. There are circumstances where other urgent concerns take precedence over confidentiality such as for mandated reporting for child abuse or neglect, for elder abuse and neglect, disabled abuse or neglect and mentally ill adult abuse and neglect. Some situations are complex such as domestic abuse, past crimes and HIV-AIDS risk behaviors and state laws differ as to reporting responsibilities that definitive guidelines cannot be responsibly provided here.

Threats of *suicide or self-harm* should always be taken seriously, and an assessment made of the possibility that the threat will be carried out; is there a specific plan, how lethal is the plan, how available is the method, and are there others in proximity that could interrupt or prevent the plan from being carried out (Bauman, 2008).

Bennett et al. (2006) suggest that mental health professionals know the procedures needed to reduce to likelihood of suicidal behavior, how these can be integrated into treatment, and the state law governing reporting responsibilities. It is very helpful to learn a systematic method for assessing suicide.

Culture and Diversity in Group Therapy

The cultural and diversity characteristics of group members can play an important role in their group participation as well as influences on interactions with other group members and the leader. Such characteristics can include but are not limited to age, race/ethnicity, national origin, language, socio-economic status, gender, sexual identity, religion, education level, occupation/career, ableness, and other cultural and diversity factors relative to the particular individual including the group leader. These characteristics affect the diagnosis, mode of therapy, transference, countertransference, and establishing the therapeutic alliance. An example of this was presented by Strakowski (2003), who found that race differences remain when diagnostic accuracy is controlled and that flawed clinical judgment can occur as a result of unawareness of cultural differences in presentation of symptoms.

These are also factors that can affect the group members, leaders, and the group itself. Among these cultural and diversity factors for all are conscious and unconscious bias and stereotyping that can lead to unintentionally insensitive remarks and statements that can affect the therapeutic relationship, and the establishment of trust and safety for the group and its members and other acts that impede the group members' growth, development, and healing. Other factors include the extent of the leader's multicultural awareness and competencies, social convention practices, and how the leader manages microaggressions.

There are some terms and concepts that may be helpful to define and/or describe for a better understanding of the possible effects they may have on the person, the group leader and on the group; culture, ethnic groups, race, acculturation, prejudice, stereotyping, multiple identities, privilege, diversity and diversity factors, intersectionality, and cultural humility.

Terms and Concepts

A *culture* is a social group that contains and transmits memories and values from one generation to the next and have distinctive customs shared among themselves. *Ethnic group* is the designation usually applied to minority groups in a culture whose members identify as different from those in the larger society, share common features, traits, religious beliefs and whose sense of identity is affected by acculturation. *Race* is defined as a group of people united or classified together on the basis of common history, nationality, or geographic distribution and who have a human genetic variation marked by specific physical characteristics common to that group. *Acculturation* is described by Alvidrez, Azocar, and Miranda (1996) as a process of psychological and social changes that occur when an individual or group is in contact with another culture., such as what happens with immigrants in the United States.

Prejudice is an irrational pattern of hostility, hatred and/or suspicion for a group of people where overgeneralizations are made on the basis of incomplete and/or inaccurate information, leading to misperceptions that negatively influence interpersonal relationships. *Stereotyping* occurs when individuals are categorized and reacted to in terms of the erroneous beliefs about that category and without acknowledgment of any exceptions to the beliefs. *Multiple identities* refer to the person's membership or characteristics that incorporate several aspects for one person such as age, gender, ableness, sexual orientation, socioeconomic status, education and profession, religion or spiritual orientation, and occupation.

Privilege provides a working definition that speaks of an invisible package of unearned assets that can be counted on to support one's position in society, or in the particular setting. *Diversity* refers to the visible and invisible characteristics that are a function of time, genetics, life circumstance, and/or personal choice, and which can contribute to perceptions and reactions of self and of others. These are characteristics such as age, gender, sexual orientation, religion, and disability. Diversity factors can also be of importance as these factors can contribute to the extent to which members are excluded or included; if they are related to as different because of visible or hidden characteristics that produce bias, stereotyping, and discrimination and the like as those could have been of importance in shaping the experiences that help form the person. These usual reactions to these diversity factors may also be played out in the group. *Intersectionality* is described by Rosenthal as:

> multiple, intersecting identities and ascribed social positions (e.g. race, gender, sexual identity, class) along with associated power dynamics, as people are at the same time members of many different social groups and have unique experiences with privilege and disadvantage because of those intersections.
>
> (Rosenthal, 2016, p. 475)

Cultural humility (Hook et al., 2013) refers to the concept that guides the group leader's perceptions and work with group members to be aware of their personal culturally embedded ideals, beliefs, and prejudices can affect their interactions with group members. It recognizes that they and group members will have a wide variety of beliefs, structures, interactional patterns and expectations (Hook et al., 2013; Ratts et al., 2016).

Culture and Diversity Awareness and Competencies

Culture and diversity factors have considerable influences on group members' development of their identity, roles, gender and sexual identity, class and status, race and ethnic identity and other self-factors are all impacted by family of origin, the community, and the larger culture. Each group member will differ in some way for each of the factors, even those that appear to be from the same community or larger culture. Group leaders will have to be especially aware and sensitive in addition to the usual group factors and individual group member factors. Fowers and Davidov (2006) propose that cultural awareness and competencies models as having three components: *awareness, knowledge,* and *skills.*

- In the *awareness component,* group leaders can become more culturally aware and competent when they examine their personal identity as a racial/cultural person, understand how their personal biases, prejudices, stereotypes, and assumptions that will impact relationships in the group, as well as the cultural differences that can impact group member.*Activity: Personal Implicit Bias Test Results*

Directions: Take the Harvard Implicit Bias Test available at no cost online. There are numerous different tests under the umbrella of Implicit Bias that have been shown to be valid and reliable and readers are encouraged to take several of these and write a brief summary of their results noting those that are surprising to them.

- The *knowledge component* includes the group leader's knowledge of the cultural influences on individual development growth, what cultural and diversity factors will impact the group members and the group process, and the leader skills that demonstrate cultural competency (Flowers & Davidov, 2007). Knowledge is also gained from other sources, such as books, articles, the internet, consultants, and so on.
- In the *skills component* there are some specific leader skills that can be developed that will promote the positive aspects of culture and diversity and also reduce their possible negative effects. The basic skills set include conveying respect and positive regard, tolerance of differences, and the basic understanding that groups become cohesive around perceived similarities and fail to do so around perceived differences.

Develop Greater Awareness and Sensitivity

Group leaders can increase their awareness and sensitivity with four steps; understand the visible differences, recognize that there are hidden differences that may be significant, and when making these visible can be helpful, engage in leader self-preparation with attention to specific leader tasks, and use strategies designed to promote knowledge, understanding and sensitivity.

Visible differences are usually the first to be noticed and highlighted But, even some of these can be misleading, and group leaders should take care to not make too many assumptions based on visible characteristics. Further, some group members may prefer that their visible differences not be emphasized, while others want some acknowledgment of these. It may be best to let the group member point out their personal differences instead of the group leader focusing on the difference. Group leaders need to also carefully examine their personal reactions to visible differences.

Indirect or hidden differences are cultural and/or diversity characteristics that are important for that person's self-identity, but these may not be visible. Examples of indirect or hidden differences that may make a difference to the person are having chronic illness, their sexual preference/orientation; values such as the role of the family; and meaning attribution for experiences derived from their culture of origin such as those being self-induced, fate or random. An indirect or hidden cultural or diversity difference may be important for one person, but not for another person with the same or similar difference. It is essential that a group leader not assume that a difference is important for a person.

Leader's self-preparation is an essential part of cultural and diversity sensitivity and competence. Group leaders will find it helpful to do some reflection about pre-conceived assumptions about culture and diversity, possible stereotypes they may have, conscious and unconscious biases and prejudices, unconscious assumptions about the value and worth of others' differences including their meaning attribution for their experiences. In addition, it would be helpful for group leaders to learn about other cultures, the impact of diversity factors on individuals, and to seek out resources such as online webinars, conferences, books and other publications and have someone to be available for consultation.

Increasing Leader's Cultural and Diversity Competence

Cultural and diversity factors are extremely important, and group leaders are encouraged to develop the needed knowledge, sensitivity, and competencies that will recognize and respect these factors. Group leaders are encouraged to keep their minds open to the many possibilities that cultural and diversity factors bring to the group, and to capitalize on these for the benefit of all group members.

It is helpful for group leaders to do and be the following.

- Not generalize about members within an ethnic/racial population but to be aware that there is considerable variation among members of the same population.
- Model respect and acceptance for diverse group members.
- Understand that it is essential to build basic trust, mutual understanding, and respect among group members before using an intervention around cultural and diversity factors.
- Demonstrate empathy, tolerance, cultural and diversity sensitivity, awareness, and knowledge.
- Develop credibility by conceptualizing members' problems in a manner congruent with their culture, but only after ascertaining what that member's culture is.
- Continue to develop personal cultural and diversity competence.

Activity: Stereotyping

Objectives: To increase awareness of possible personal stereotypes, to clarify stereotypes held about particular groups.

Materials: Five 3" × 5" index cards, a pen or pencil for each participant, masking tape, and five prepared large sheets of newsprint each having one of the following words or phrases: Homeless; Bipolar; Single mother; Rich unemployed female; Parolee.

Procedure:

1 Using the masking tape, post the newsprint with the words or phrases and distribute the index cards and pens or pencils.
2 Ask participants to write the posted words and phrases on the cards, one to a card.
3 Instruct participants to write all the stereotypes they've heard for each word and phrase.
4 Ask participants to then walk around the room and write their stereotypes for each word or phrase, but to not repeat any.
5 Discuss the stereotypes that were written.

References

AGPA & IBCGP. (2002). *Guidelines for Ethics in Group Psychotherapy*. New York: American Group Psychotherapy Association & International Board of Certified Group Psychotherapists.

Alvidrez, J., Azocar, F., & Miranda, J. (1996). Demystifying the concept of ethnicity for psychotherapy researchers. *Journal of Consulting and Clinical Psychology*, 64 (5), 903–908. doi:10.1037/0022-006X.64.5.903.

Bauman, S. (2008). *Essential Topics for the Helping Professional*. Boston, MA: Allyn & Bacon.

Bennett, B., *et al.* (2006). *Assessing and Managing Risk in Psychological Practice*. Rockville, MD: The Trust.

Brown, N. (2009). *Becoming a Group Leader*. Upper Saddle River, NJ: Pearson Education.

Brown, N. (2019). *Conducting Effective Psychoeducational Groups*. New York: Routledge.

Fowers, B. J., & Davidov, B. J. (2006). The virtue of multiculturalism: Personal transformation, character, and openness to the other. *American Psychologist*, 61(6), 581–594. doi:10.1037/0003-066X.61.6.581.

Hook, J. N., Davis, D. E., Owen, J., Worthington, E. L., & Utsey, S. O. (2013). Cultural humility: Measuring openness to culturally diverse clients. *Journal of Counseling Psychology*, 60(3), 353–366. doi:10.1037/a0032595.

Lilenfeld, S. (2007). Psychological treatments that cause harm. *Perspectives on Psychological Science*, 2, 53–70.

MacNair-Semands, R. (2015). *Ethics in Group Therapy*. New York: AGPA.

Ratts, M., Singh, A., Nassar-McMillan, S., & Butler, S. (2016). Multicultural and social justice counseling competencies: Guidelines for the counseling profession. *Journal of Multicultural counseling and Development*, 44(1), 28–48. doi:10.1002/jmcd.12035.

Rosenthal, L. (2016). Incorporating intersectionality into psychology: An opportunity to promote social justice and equity. *American Psychologist*, 71(6), 474–485. doi:10.1037/a0040323.

Strakowski, S. (2003). How to avoid ethnic bias when diagnosing schizophrenia. *Current Psychiatry*, 2(6), 72–82.

Tuckman, B. W. (1965). Development sequence in small groups. *Psychological Bulletin*, 63(6), 384–399.

6 Therapeutic Components for Groups

Group Therapeutic Factors

Teaching how to implement group therapeutic factors can be a challenge as some are intangible and not easy to describe, identify and to help emerge in the group. The following presentation will first present some information and evidence for the importance and efficacy for each factor which can be used for lectures and digital presentations, examples for identification, suggestions for helping the factor to emerge, suggestions for embedding self-development in the lectures, and guides for using discussions or case studies or activities. The specific therapeutic factors presented are based on those presented by Yalom and Leszcz (2021), and while there may be other such factors, the presentation will also help instructors decide how to present those.

Universality highlights similarities among group members which helps to reduce feelings of alienation and isolation, promote feelings of belonging and inclusion, and reduce fears. An added benefit for universality is that it helps to develop cohesion groups become cohesive around similarities and stay disconnected and detached around differences. Agazarian (1997)

What may be of more importance for universality are other not-so-visible similarities, such as past experiences, values, emotional reactions, needs, desires and fantasies. Any of these, when made visible, can help forge connections at a deeper and more meaningful level.

Tip: Link similarities for members around experiences, values, interests, and other meaningful commonalties. Do not highlight differences but acknowledge when members highlight their difference that this difference is important for them.

Existential factors are cited by Yalom (1980) and Yalom and Leszcz (2021) as therapeutic for group members, as emerging during the life span of the group, sometimes in an obvious way and sometimes in indirect and disguised ways and are often overlooked or minimized. Some major existential factors that can emerge in the group are meaning and purpose in life, emptiness, pain and suffering, isolation and alienation, freedom and responsibility, existential anxiety, and the inevitability of death.

Some members enter group with issues around *meaning and purpose* in their lives. These members will say that they feel empty and unfulfilled.

DOI: 10.4324/9781003329787-6

From the outside they have full lives, but they report that much of what they do seems meaningless.

Tip: Guide the member(s) in accepting that they are the only ones who can determine what is meaningful and purposeful for them.

Emptiness has nothing as its primary state. There seems to be nothing at the core of the person, and they will report feeling hollow, having a hole, unable to feel intensely. Activities, drugs, alcohol, and other self-defeating acts can be their ways of trying to feel less empty.

Tip: The group leader's task is to block other group members from giving advice on how to feel less empty instead, ask them to describe what they do so as to not feel empty.

One of the first things almost every group member seeks and wants is relief from their *pain and suffering*. However, this is not possible and most members need and want some hope that one day there will be relief. The existential piece is that pain and suffering is a human condition and, although some relief is possible for some people at some time, there will continue to be pain and suffering throughout one's life.

Tip: Help members understand that pain and suffering are universal, is a part of the human condition, and happens to everyone at some time.

The existential concerns of *alienation and isolation* occur when people do not feel that they can connect with others. There is something within that is making them feel that they are different and not allowing them to reach out to others. Or, they can feel that they are being excluded and not being welcomed to connect. Either way, the lack of meaningful human connections is troubling.

Tip: Teach and show them how to reach out to others in the group to develop connections.

The ability to make personal choices, to decide for oneself, and to develop one's capacity is one way of conceptualizing *freedom*. The other side of freedom is responsibility as one cannot be an authentic human without also assuming responsibility.

Reflection: Ask group members to reflect on how choices are overlooked or ignored. To consider when events, circumstances and other people intervened to direct or even select the choice for them. Even when they could have made a conscious choice, they did not make the choice, that, although they have or had choices, they do or did not always make the decision what or what not to do.

One of the more terrifying things many humans face is the awareness of their *death*. Ceasing to be is so upsetting that they will do almost anything to keep from accepting that one day they will cease to exist. Thus, almost everyone goes out of their way to avoid even the thought of death. However much the idea of death is avoided or ignored, it still appears in the group.

Tip: Ask members to reflect and describe ways of being dead in the group and how that feels. Examples include withdrawal, refusal to connect, lack of responding to others.

Hope is defined here as the individual's inner encouragement and support (Brown, 2002). Hope is unique for each group member, and members may not even be able to describe what can trigger their hopefulness. Hope does not deny or minimize the reality of the individual's experiencing or predicament, nor does it seek to perceive these through "rose-colored glasses" (Davis, 1999; Elliott, 1997; Hopper, 2001).

Tip: Explore with members their hopes for what the group will do for them and how they can make their hopes realistic and accomplished.

Altruism is defined as a concern for the welfare of others that is selfless. That is, the giver does not expect gratitude, liking, joining, or reciprocity. The concern is a gift with no strings attached (Brown, 2002). Hafen et al. (1996) notes that altruism has been termed as one of the healthiest characteristics that humans can possess. There are studies linking altruism to health, counteracting stress and bolstering the immune system.

Tip: Ask members to reflect on how they feel when they receive altruistic acts, such as unexpected kindness, a response that shows that they were understood and valued, and so on.

Family of Origin Factors include parental relationships, sibling relationship and other family issues. Families are where members receive the foundation for their growth and development. The interaction of genetic predispositions, environment, and basic personality are significant factors with family falling under environmental factors. The individual's position and role in the family, how they were interacted with, the relationships with parents and siblings, early relationship deprivations and so on, all have an impact on their growth and development.

Catharsis can also be described as emotional venting.so that tension and anxiety from suppressed and denied feelings are relieved. There are times when just speaking of feelings that are being held in is sufficient, but Yalom (1980) and Yalom and Leszcz (2021) note that this is of limited value if some intrapersonal learning does not accompany the catharsis. *Interpersonal learning* occurs with feedback from other group members. Members can also experiment with new behavior in the group that can lead to improved relationships outside the group. How members relate to the leader and other group members mirrors how they relate to people outside the group, especially those who are in close or intimate relationships with them. The in-group behavior will differ in quality and intensity, but will be basically the same. *Socializing techniques* can be a helpful benefit for group members and can help reduce or eliminate isolation and alienation. Members can become more aware of their characteristic relating styles, the reception and impact this style has on others, and practice new behaviors that can be more constructive.

Imitative behavior is when group members learn from the modeling behavior of the group leader and from other group members. It is important for the group leader to have a heightened awareness of what they are doing, what the behavior reflects about their inner state, and what is being communicated to group members. Members learn much from observing the group leader and this learning can be from behavior that is intentional or unintentional, or conscious or unconscious on their part. This is another reason why the personal development of the group leader is critical to prevent unintentional communications. *Imparting information* is an integral part of many groups to clarify misunderstandings, correct factual errors, understand a process, learning where other needed information can be found, attain new knowledge, and can assist in decision making. *Group cohesiveness* allows and encourages group member to work effectively and efficiently on group and individual goals, members are appreciative of the resources of the group, interpersonal learning is facilitated as members feel safer and are more trusting, and members are taking more risks and responsibility for their growth and development.

Fundamental Relationship Attributes

The basic relationship attributes needed as a group leader are essentially the same as those needed for individual therapy but may need to be used in a different way. For example, attending is used in both individual and group therapy. In group, the leader needs to attend to all members in the group and stay in touch with the group-as-a-whole, not just the person who is talking. Fundamental relationship attitudes are genuineness, caring, positive regard, respect, and acceptance.

Being authentic or *genuine* is essential when establishing the therapeutic relationship. It is infinitely more difficult to mask or fake attitudes in a group, especially since members are paying very close attention to you. Being real and authentic in your attitudes and behaviors is important to build trust between you and members, and to encourage disclosures about very shameful and painful personal information. Can you fool someone into believing you are genuine when you are not? Yes, you can. But, on some level, the other person knows you are faking. You do not want to pretend to have an attitude you do not have if you expect group members to trust you enough to reveal secrets they may never have talked about to anyone before. Deceit does not build trust in a relationship.

The leader can promote feelings of trust and safety by making members feel *cared for* and that they are held in *positive regard*. Group members must develop feelings of safety and trust in the leader and group before they can conquer their fears enough to allow themselves to talk about sensitive issues and concerns. Many members enter group feeling guilty, ashamed, and afraid that they will be perceived by the leader and, other group members, as bad and fatally flawed. Many fear rejection and destruction if their "real self" were to be revealed. However, letting the "real self" be known is helpful if healing is to take place, behaviors and/or attitudes changed, or growth and development to occur. On the one hand, members must reveal their shamed "self", and on the other hand, revealing it is feared to have dire consequences. What a leader does and says is critical to providing a group atmosphere to encourage self-disclosure and overcome fears.

Positive regard and *respect* for others are intertwined. Positive regard is more a part of who you are and your basic view of human nature. Respect is also internal to some extent but has external manifestations that convey to the other person that you do, or do not, respect them.

You have to be able to regard others as worthwhile unique individuals in order to respect them. They are separate, different, and no less worthy than anyone else. They have positive characteristics, flaws, failings, and potentials; and you remain aware that each person has something to contribute.

Respect, caring and positive regard all contribute to being able to *accept* group members as they are. Yes, they have issues, problems and concerns; and yes, they are there to get help and change, but before any of this can take place, members have to feel that they are accepted. This acceptance builds trust for the leader and the group.

Accepting group members as they are can also contribute to the therapeutic group factor of hopefulness. When the leader can be aware of group members' problems, etc., and not dismiss or write them off as hopeless, members can "catch" the leader's attitude that there is hope that they can and will resolve their problems, overcome their concerns, and/or work through their issues. Do not underestimate the importance of this factor or the contribution acceptance can make to the group and to individual group members. Eye contact can be used to show interest in the other person, but if there is no real interest, your eye contact can become glazed and, on some level, the person knows that you are not interested.

Responding or Communication Competencies

Responding or communication competencies are divided into two categories: basic and fundamental skills used in individual and group counseling, and skills that have a particular application to group leadership. While the therapeutic relationship is important, it is not sufficient to promote work in the group. The leader also has to be competent and use responding skills that promote the development of safety and trust, encourage members to self-disclose, promote interaction among members, model more effective communications and recognition of emotional investment for members, and that direct a focus to important content and feelings for both individual members and for the group as a whole.

Basic competencies include active listening and responding, appropriate questioning, a focus on personal experiencing of members, encouraging direct responses among members, redirecting and reframing.

Listening and Responding

It is essential that group leaders hone their listening skills as the ability to hear what is said, what is meant, and understand the underlying feelings is crucial to helping group members. Listening in a group setting is considerably more difficult than in an individual session as the interactions are faster and more complex. Listening is basic to empathizing, confronting and re-directing. Content may be important however, the feelings carry the most important part of the message. Hearing the content allows you to make hypotheses about the feeling the person may not be expressing (Rutan, 1993). Listening and responding is discussed more fully with examples and strategies in the section on empathy.

Questioning

Knowing when to probe and how to probe so as not to make the receiver feel attacked or become defensive is a skill that can be learned. The most important aspect of this skill is learning when not to ask questions. Brown (1998) lists three basic uses for questioning; to obtain data and information, to clarify misunderstandings, and to pinpoint something in order to take immediate action (pp. 52–53).

The group leader should be especially careful not to ask numerous questions and to refrain from focusing on a member and pelting them with questions, even if that person is talking about something where considerable clarification is needed. Refrain from asking questions where possible as some people can have a negative response to being questioned. Trotzer (1989) notes that most questions are statements that signal what the speaker wants, especially questions that are used as probes to guide the receiver to areas the speaker feels important.

The following are less useful and should either not be used, or used sparingly: limiting questions, hot seat questions, hypothetical questions, disguised demands, masked needs, and rhetorical questions (Brown, 1998).

Limiting and hypothetical questions may have some small value. For example, limiting questions force members to make a choice from a few options. Hypothetical questions could allow for some creative brainstorming to take place by posing a "what if" scenario. Some questions are *disguised demands*. Instead of directly asking for what is wanted, the person tries to manipulate the other person by asking a question. Another way that questions are not direct communication is when they are used to *mask needs*. The person wants or needs something but, instead of saying what he/she wants or needs, a question is substituted. *Rhetorical* questions are questions to which there are no answers, or to which the answers are already known. Neither is useful to facilitate communication, understanding, or the relationship. There are two instances where questions can be helpful and constructive gathering facts and initiating clarifications. It is also helpful for the group leader to block questioning by group members especially where statements and empathic responding could be made.

Direct Responses

If the leader will model speaking and responding directly to group members, then members will most likely follow that example. Responding directly includes attending to the speaker, to first reflect what was heard, to not go off on a tangent no matter how much the tangent is related, acknowledging their perspective. This is valuable in communicating even when your next statement shows that you disagree or have a different viewpoint.

Other ways of being direct are to openly express important feelings as they are experienced in the interactions, giving constructive feedback, not suppressing important feelings for fear of alienating someone, and by being patient when they are talking and not interrupting. Directness begins with the non-verbal attending behaviors. Always orient your body toward the person, become present centered, and maintain eye contact. Try to not be distracted, and be willing to express your important feelings, when appropriate. It may not always be appropriate for you to openly express your feelings and you need to learn to judge when you should and when it will be best for all concerned if you do not. For example, it will probably not be wise to express your anger openly and directly in the beginning stages of group.

Practice paraphrasing and reflecting so that they become an integral part of your communication style. It may seem somewhat artificial and redundant when you first begin to use these skills, but you will find that you will reduce misunderstandings and miscommunications and most importantly, you will make the receiver feel valued and respected. Group members will find this an invaluable skill that has implications for their relationships outside the group.

Reframing and Redirecting

Reframing and redirecting are also termed re-labeling and noted as a positive group leadership skill by Agazarian, (1997). Reframing occurs when you repeat to the group member what he/she said giving it another perspective. The change is a different way to say whatever was said. For example, if the member noted that conflict was upsetting and she could never be comfortable with it, a reframe could be noting that she prefers that her relationships be harmonious.

Reframing is most useful when the speaker's statements are focused on deficiencies, weaknesses or mistakes whether personal or directed at other members; a member fails to perceive positive aspects of the situation or of his/her effectiveness, when a member cannot see personal strengths, and/or when the speaker has a negative perspective, such as hopelessness, and another perspective could provide hope. The important thing to remember about reframing is that you do not change the content, as that could distort the original meaning. The reframe points out current experiencing, how it could be viewed differently, and opens the door for consideration that there are other possibilities.

Redirecting is similar to reframing except that in this case, you are actively asking the person to go in another direction. You, as the leader, have noted something you consider important that is being missed, ignored, overlooked, or minimized by the speaker and/or the group. Reframing is generally used with individual group members while redirecting can be used with both individuals and the group-as-a-whole. It is particularly effective when used at the group level.

Group Process and Process Illumination

Process refers to the relationship being expressed in the here and now (Brown, 2003). The relationship may be between individuals, between subgroups, or between the group and the leader. Although reasons for expression of the relationship may have antecedents from past relationships, such as parental, or from past experiences, the focus for using process relies on here and now expressing. The focus and emphasis are on what is taking place in the group at the present time, not why.

Highlighting process tends to promote understanding for both personal individual issues, and for group issues. Chapman (1971) proposes that "personality consists of the relatively long-term ways in which a person engages in interpersonal relationships" and "can be studied, understood and sometimes changed only in the context of interpersonal relationships". Observing interpersonal relationships in the group provides a mechanism for some understanding of what life experiences have formed the individual. We can only speculate about the nature and quality of the person's early relationships as we only have the present interpersonal relationships with which to work, and the person's recollections and feelings about their early relationships, which are generally flawed.

Process commentary can focus on what is happening between group members, or in the group-as-a-whole. Some unconscious, non-conscious, and unspoken relationships between members that can form the basis for process commentary are the following:

- Members seeking to connect.
- Attempts to dominate or control.
- Solicitation of support or approval.
- Rejection.
- A need to take care of others.
- Avoiding intimacy.
- Yearning for fusion.

Some unspoken needs or desires for the group-as-a-whole are safety, trust, resistance, aggression, fear of engulfment, fear of exclusion, depression, clarification of norms, feelings of helplessness, or fear of destruction. Once you identify what the needs are, this forms the basis for your process commentary.

Since it is considerably more difficult to make group-as-a-whole process commentary, this discussion will present information to guide you in understanding when process is important to illuminate, how to tune in to process, and guidelines for making commentary. The most important points to remember are that the primary responsibility for making process commentary lies with the group leader, and process commentary is effective when an issue critical to the existence or functioning of the entire group takes precedence over individual issues. It is also helpful to remember that what is taking place in the group is also reflective of what is taking place for members, although their experiencing may be different.

Indices of Process

How does the leader identify process for the group-as-a-whole? What are some indicators? These questions, and others, are difficult to answer in definitive terms as process is ever present, changing and about as substantial as fog. The group leader is very busy tuning in to the dynamics in the group, needs of individual group members, objectives for the sessions and goals for the group, as well as the leader's personal experiencing on both the cognitive and affective levels. Further, identification of process is very complex and a group leader develops confidence in their ability to tune in to process over time. While it can be helpful to observe a group leader making process commentary and receiving explanations of the basis for the comments, the only way to learn is to practice identifying process and making commentary.

It is difficult at first, to focus on the group. Most group leaders first develop their skills with individuals and tend to want to focus exclusively on individuals in the group. Focusing on and intervening with individuals is productive, but until group members learn how to coat-tail that is, use what you are doing with one individual to work on their personal issues, the leader is not doing group therapy or group counseling but rather is doing individual therapy in a group setting. Group therapy and group counseling that use the resources of the group to help individuals is very effective and allows all members to work at the same time. Making group level process commentary allows the leader to work with all group members.

Some specific indices that indicate that there may be a need for group process commentary are the following.

- Behaviors of the group, what the group is doing, or is not doing.
- Feelings generated in the leader.
- Similar feelings noted in members from their nonverbal behavior, but not verbalized by them.
- The negative impact of some behavior on members.
- Links between members' issues, concerns, and feelings.

- Themes that emerge in group.
- When the group becomes mired or stuck.

There are four assumptions that guide this discussion on process and process commentary.

1   There are numerous effective ways to respond or intervene; some are more effective than others.
2   An important source of information about the group and what is happening are the leader's reactions and feelings. Learning to access these and use the information takes a high degree of self- awareness, self-knowledge, and a willingness to confront personal countertransference.
3   Some responses and/or interventions are made at the group level, others to individuals. Both are important and crucial.
4   In order to know what is going on in the group you have to observe the dynamics. Developing the expertise to tune in and identify important dynamics at the moment takes time and effort. Practice, with feedback, aids in developing expertise.

Leader Tasks and Skills

Since the primary responsibility for process commentary lies with the leader, there are certain tasks and skills that the leader must develop and use. These tasks and skills include all of the following.

- Assuming a present-centered focus.
- Containing the group's anxiety, fears, rage, and other emotions, without becoming overwhelmed.
- Understand group dynamics.
- Teach members to assume a process orientation by learning to accept process illumination remarks.
- Use the expected behaviors for the stage of group as a guide for understanding what the group is experiencing when using process commentary.
- Provide constructive feedback.
- Be judicious in use of process commentary.

Use a Present-Centered Focus

The skill of immediacy will be of great help in the ability to have a present-centered focus when making process commentary. It is easier to reflect on what is taking place and think about what to do, but you do not have the time to come back the next session, or even later in this session, to decide to make the commentary. In order to be effective, process commentary must occur as close to the time when the behaviors were observed as possible.

A major premise for group level process commentary is that whatever the group is doing or discussing, it is always talking about itself and is a reflection of what is taking place in the group. Another premise is that behavior of any group member at any time is reflective of personal needs, history, behavior patterns and of the group's needs, history, behavior patterns etc. Focusing on the present and making it visible helps both the group and individual members.

Observe what is being done and what is being avoided or resisted, and what behaviors are expected for the particular stage of group development. This forms a basis for your commentary. In addition it is helpful to use the present tense when phrasing process commentary. It is more difficult for group members to deny observable behavior that takes place in the here and now, and to resist. Process commentary is more likely to be accepted when you do this because there has not been an intervening period where events could be forgotten or distorted. Resistance is also lessened because the leader does not make inferences about motivation, but only highlights what is taking place at that time. While members are free to accept or reject the process commentary, they are more likely to accept it and work with it because of the immediacy.

The Leader as a Container

The leader who uses process must be aware of their ability to function as the container for the group's most uncomfortable feelings, such as fear or rage. This is one reason why it is crucial for the leader to be able to tune in to his/her current experiencing as this experiencing most often provides clues or data about what the group is experiencing. For example, if you as the leader find yourself experiencing fear or dread and the group continues to discuss outside concerns, it is likely that you are containing the group's fear of establishing relationships, intimacy, and so on, although you identify your feeling as dread.

Group members use the leader and the group to contain primitive affects, such as rage and fear, and to defend against experiencing anxiety, shame, and guilt. Most often, the leader has to be the container for the group so that feelings of safety and trust can be established, members do not feel overwhelmed by affect, control of intense affect can be maintained, and modeling of effective ways of dealing with intense emotions can occur.

Identify the Group Dynamics

The ability to identify group dynamics aids in understanding process and making process commentary. Group dynamics define the process taking place and provide the mechanics or structure for identifying and understanding process. Basic dynamics are: levels of participation, communication patterns, resistances, nonverbal communication, and feelings aroused and expressed or not expressed.

The leader uses current experiencing and observation of group dynamics in focusing on process. What are members doing or not doing, saying or avoiding, how are feelings being expressed or suppressed, what do nonverbal behaviors signal, changes in levels of participation, communication patterns and changes are some dynamics that can be observed and used. The leader would use the dynamics for the group as a whole to better understand both what the group is experiencing and what members are experiencing.

Groups go through stages of development although the stage of development the group is currently in is sometimes hard to determine. Transition points are not definitive. Further, if the group is an open group and new members added at any time, the group regresses in some ways and stages become even more difficult to distinguish. Most groups, both open and closed, do move through stages. Review the material in chapter four for more suggestions on how to use this information.

Teaching Members

A continuing task for group leaders is to teach members to accept process commentary. Members have to learn how to assume a process orientation that is, tuning in to the process as well as their personal thoughts and feelings. This is not an easy task and a group leader needs to realize and accept that it will take time before members are comfortable with process commentary.

It may be helpful to explain to members that you will make group-as-a-whole comments, especially when linking members' concerns or issues, addressing an impasse, when the discussion becomes stuck or circular, and when the group appears to be resisting. There will also be times when you will make process commentary about what seems to be happening between individual members or between you and the group. Assure members that they do not have to agree with your comments but, if they do take exception to them to say so directly and be willing to work on any differences in perception with you in the group. No outside meetings should be used for this.

The most helpful characteristic for a group leader to possess when teaching members to accept process commentary is patience. Do not expect members to be comfortable at first with either your comments on process, or when they openly disagree with you. After all, in the beginning stages of group the leader is expected to be all knowing and all powerful and members are reluctant to openly disagree.

Process Commentary as Constructive Feedback

Leaders generally consider all their feedback to be constructive. However, when feedback is interpretative it tends to be perceived as threatening by members instead of constructive. Members tend to hear old parental messages of blame and criticism awakening shame and guilt when interpretations are made. These perceptions and reactions are the main reasons why process commentary should limit interpretation and be given in a way that reduces defensiveness and resistance. It should be presented so that it increases willingness to accept the comment. Process commentary is not helpful if you then have to work through defensiveness and resistance. Group leaders that use constructive feedback take into account the emotional needs of members, limit feedback to that which is of most importance for the functioning of the group, links together commonalities of group members, can be tied to observable behavior(s), and do not couch the feedback in terms that bestow blame or criticism.

Even when members become accepting of process commentary, a group leader should not overuse it. Group level interventions are very helpful and seem to address individual members' concerns as well as the group-as-a-whole issues. Members learn how they contribute to conditions such as group resistance and how to accept responsibility for the group's condition, such as suppression of anger, leading to self-exploration of how this behavior in group reflects their behavior outside of group.

Process commentary can arouse intense feelings, trigger old parental messages, tap in to shame and guilt feelings, and strengthen defensiveness and resistance. These are reasons why the group leader should reserve process commentary for those times when highlighting and emphasizing process would promote understanding, resolve an impasse, or highlight progress.

Process Commentary Skills

There are characteristics and skills needed to be an effective group leader and many of these also apply to making process commentary. Characteristics such as warmth, caring, positive regard, acceptance and genuineness all contribute to establishing trust and safety in the group as well as confidence in the group leader. These characteristics are fundamental in helping group members accept process commentary.

Skills such as immediacy, concreteness, reflection, active listening and responding, and linking can be refined to provide effective process commentary. Other skills, such as timing, are developed as a result of experience and cannot be taught or adequately defined to provide specific guidelines or steps.

Immediacy, as a skill, refers to the here and now part of the commentary. This means that the group leader phrases the comment to focus on what is taking place in the present. The present may be defined as the entire session, a portion of the session, or even an event that is currently taking place. While there may be other related events in the past that can be tied to current experiencing, the most effective process commentary uses current events. Further, resistance is much less when the comment focuses on observable behavior (i.e. can stand up to consensual validation by group members).

Concreteness is helpful because it does not infer motives or make judgments. Again, observable behavior is the focus. This is what group members are doing or saying, not what someone infers. It is helpful when the leader can describe specific behaviors or label their personal feelings. If there are several behaviors; such as several members use the same word, term or phrase, that can be pointed out as part of the description; be specific about what was said or done. If the leader is using their personal feelings as clues to group process, then label these feelings and accept responsibility for them. Say very clearly that these are your feelings about what is taking place. Give members some wiggle room just in case accepting the process commentary is too threatening at the present moment.

Reflection is probably the most useful skill of all because it holds a mirror up to a member or the group without blaming, criticizing, or judging. Simple reflective statements can be very powerful in encouraging or forcing members to examine what they are saying, doing and feeling. While the leader may understand why they are acting this way, or certain feelings were triggered, there is no need to report this information at this time. It is much more effective to simply reflect, allow members to self-examine, and come to these understandings on their own. By doing so, defensiveness and resistance are reduced, or more easily worked through.

Active listening and responding speaks of the hidden messages that the feelings are communicating. These useful skills highlight expressed and unexpressed feelings in the group. Highlighting feelings aids the group in coming to grips with their emotions. Members may be unfamiliar with awareness of current feelings, openly expressing them, methods they use to block feelings of self and others, or of soothing behavior and process commentary points out what they are doing and the impact of the behavior.

Linking is a very valuable group leadership skill. Tying together feelings and behavior, commonalties among members, and current and past experiences or events are ways by which members gain awareness and understanding of their issues and how the group begins to become cohesive. Linking is also the way in which a leader can know the emerging, or emerged, group theme that is defining underlying issues being worked on in the group. These underlying issues may be very different from presenting problems or expressed objectives. Making them known or visible promotes progress for the group and members.

There are several ways to link, and a group leader may use any or all of them. One way is to use the feeling works expressed by members and tie them together. For example, if group members express irritation, feelings of being devalued or criticized even though members are using outside events as the vehicle for these feelings, the leader can link them to highlight members' unspoken feelings about the group.

Another way is for the leader to use free association. This calls for a high degree of self-awareness on the part of the leader as well as the ability to think fast. To free associate you allow thoughts and feelings about what is happening to emerge until you can discern a pattern that leads to some understanding of the process to the point where you can feel comfortable making a process commentary.

Sometimes when the leader is functioning as a container for the more uncomfortable feelings for the group, you can sort through those feelings and link them to events in the group. You then are expressing the unexpressed feelings as well as helping members understand how they are avoiding, suppressing, or projecting feelings in the group that, in turn, can be linked to characteristic behaviors outside the group.

References

Agazarian, Y. (1997) *Systems-Centered Therapy for Groups*. New York: The Guilford Press.

Brown, N. (1998). *The Destructive Narcissistic Pattern*. Westport, CT: Praeger.

Brown, N. (2002). *Whose Life Is it Anyway?*. Oakland, CA: New Harbinger Publishers.

Brown, N. (2003). *Psychoeducational Groups* (2nd ed.). New York: Taylor & Francis.

Chapman, J. (1971). Development and validation of a scale to measure empathy. *Journal of Counseling Psychology*, 18(3), 281–282.

Davis, N. (1999). *Resilience: Status of the Research and Research Based Programs*. Draft working paper. Bethesda MD: Substance Abuse and Mental Health Services administration, Center for Mental Health Services, Division of Program Development Special Populations & Projects, Special Programs Development Branch.

Elliott, D. M. (1997). Traumatic events: Prevalence and delayed recall in the general population. *Journal of Consulting and Clinical Psychology*, 65, 811–820.

Hafen, B. Q., Karren, K. J., Frandsen, K. J., & Smith, N. L. (1996). *Mind/Body Health*. Boston, MA: Allyn and Bacon.

Hopper, E. (2001). On the nature of hope in psychoanalysis and group analysis. *British Journal of Psychotherapy*, 18(2), 1–21.

Rogers, C. (1951). *Client-Centered Therapy*. Boston: Houghton Mifflin.

Rogers, C. (1970). *On Encounter Groups*. New York: Harper & Row.

Rutan, J. S. (1993). Psychoanalytic group psychotherapy. In H. I. Kaplan & B. J. Saddock (Eds.), *Comprehensive Group Therapy* (3rd edition, pp. 98–150). Baltimore, MD: Williams & Wilkins.

Trotzer, J. P. (1989). *The Counselor and the Group: Integrating Theory, Training and Practice* (2nd edition). Muncie, IN: Accelerated Development.

Yalom, I. (1980) *Existential Psychotherapy*. New York: Basic Books.

Yalom, I. & Leszcz, M. (2021). *The Theory and Practice of Group Psychotherapy* (6th edition). New York: Basic Books.

7 Constructive Uses of the Therapeutic Self

Therapeutic Attunement

Therapeutic attunement is a necessary part of establishing the therapeutic alliance, and is central for identifying, preventing, and intervening with problems. Aron (1996) proposes that healing is facilitated when there is optimal therapeutic attunement to the other's experiencing. Livingston and Livingston (1998) use the term "empathic attunement" (p. 382) to describe how the group leader can become aware of members' vulnerability during those times when the self of the member is unprotected and may be in danger of experiencing shame, humiliation, or fragmentation. Wright (2000) uses silent countertransference in much the same way when he writes, "The assumptions are that, first, countertransference can be induced by the client and, second, by examining it the therapist may better understand the patient's internal experience." (p. 185) Others, such as Stolorow (1993), Beebe and Lachmann (1998), and Cohen (2000), describe therapeutic attunement and its deepening and curative aspects.

When members experience vulnerable moments, this can present an opportunity for positive learning experiences for the affected member(s), and for the entire group (Livingston & Livingston, 1998). Vulnerable moments are the fleeting times where defenses are lowered, and the person is "open, available and tender" (p. 23). It is the moment where the group leader can deepen the experience to promote a genuine understanding of the member's pain and vulnerability, promote "empathic resonance" (p. 26). This is one way that the corrective emotional experience occurs, and empathic failures are repaired Yalom (1995). The responsiveness and emotional availability of the group leader is critical to this process. Therapeutic attunement can be particularly useful in understanding difficult groups where the problem remains obscure for the leader.

Empathy is a central and essential component for establishing a therapeutic alliance/ relationship as are identifying and repairing empathic failures and these topics are discussed in more detail in Chapter 8.

DOI: 10.4324/9781003329787-7

Developing a Therapeutic Alliance

Norcross & Lambert (2018), Constantino et al. (2018), Elliott et al. (2018), and Flückiger et al. (2018) all report that the working alliance, empathy and expectations are the main components of therapeutic change. Other factors that related to the psychotherapeutic relationship and change include, collaboration, collaborative goal setting, positive regard and affirmation, the therapist's empathy and using feedback. Ardito and Rabellino (2011) reviewed the relationship between the therapeutic alliance and outcomes and found that the quality of the client-therapist alliance to be a reliable predictor of positive clinical outcomes. Wampold and Imel (2015) describes the benefits of the therapeutic relationship are derived from an empathic trusting relationship, from the client's belief in the treatment's efficacy to achieve the therapeutic goals, and their actions that promote healing and change.

Bordin (1979) proposed a definition of therapeutic alliance that has three important components; a collaborative agreement for the goals of treatment and for the tasks involved in the treatment, and that both the therapist and client have positive feelings about each other. This definition gives the responsibility for treatment and outcomes to both the group leader and the group member as both have to believe in the efficacy of the chosen treatment as well as a belief that the group leader has the ability to provide effective treatment. Ardito and Rabellino (2011) stated that the quality of the therapeutic alliance is a reliable predictor of favorable treatment outcomes regardless of the psychotherapy approach.

The therapeutic alliance group leaders establish with members relies on the group leader's essential self (as discussed in Chapter 3) to be seen as trustworthy, and as competent to care for the members. Members have to feel protected, cared for, valued, understood, accepted, and perceived as worthwhile before they feel they will not be destroyed or harmed when disclosing painful material. Trusting and feeling safe is a process that unfolds as group members observe and interact with the group leader and other group members. It is unlikely that group members begin the group trusting and feeling safe.

The group leader can reassure members as much as they want to, but that reassurance will not convince members that they should trust and feel safe. Wampold and Imel (2015) describe the Rogerian conditions of warmth, acceptance, caring, concern, positive regard, tolerance and being non-judgmental as basic therapist's attributes. Group leaders will find it beneficial to be genuinely warm, caring, accepting, and act in accordance with their personality, and values rather than just using a set of techniques.

Tip: There are some nonverbal behaviors, such as maintaining eye contact and orienting your body to the speaker, learning and using group members' names, and empathic responding that can help convey these qualities to members, and you are encouraged to develop and use these.

It is important to realize is that, although these nonverbal behaviors can be observed, if the leader is not "real" or authentic, there will group members who will discern the falseness underlying the nonverbal behavior. They will, in turn, feel the falseness and be wary. Thus, it will be difficult or almost impossible to build sufficient trust and safety in the group.

Tip: Build an inner therapeutic self (as described in Chapter 3) so that these attributes become a a integral part of how of yourself and not just a technique to be used in a therapy session. This incorporation and integration will allow reactions without having to always consciously analyze before deciding what to do.

Establishing Safety

The concept of feeling psychologically safe is individualistic, and not easy to define for that reason. Group members, no matter their ages, come to group with varying degrees of the ability to tolerate intimacy, fears of being destroyed or abandoned, having experienced events that have left them cautious, and with painful associations as well as the presenting problems that have unique qualities for each person. Members may not have a good understanding of what their psychological safety needs are, much less be willing to openly express these. When group leaders rush to give members what they feel that group members need to feel psychologically safe, they can be acting based on their countertransference, and may be fueling even more uncertainty for them as feeling safe can differ from the leader and from that for other group members.

For example, suppose as the leader you feel safer when you are verbally reassured you are doing it right, and then begin to respond to each member with the kind of verbal reassurance you would want. What can happen is that some members will feel less safe. These reassurances will resonate with members who have needs similar to yours, but not all members have that need. Your reassurances may appear off-target, patronizing, unresponsive to any member who has a different need. This is why group leaders have to have sufficient personal development so that they know what their needs are, and that they are responding to what members' need, not satisfying a personal need.

Promoting Trust

Members also arrive at group with varying levels of trust for others. The group leader has the task of building trust, not only trust for the group leader, but also among group members. What a group leader generally encounters is a collection of people who do not trust them, or other members, and in some cases, do not trust themselves.

Before the group can become a place where members will risk revealing secrets, innermost thoughts and feelings, deep fears, or recall of painful events; they will have to have sufficient trust. Trust means that they come to believe that they will not be rejected, unfairly evaluated, destroyed, abandoned, ridiculed, or perceived as weak or inadequate by the leader and/or other members. This is a crucial task for the group leader because the work will stay on the surface if members do not disclose important material.

Regardless of how trustworthy the group leader may consider themselves to be, they cannot expect members to trust them just because they want and expect to be trusted, or because the leader reassures group members that they can be trusted. Trust takes time to develop, and may be especially difficult for group members who have experiences many instances where they trusted someone and was disappointed or betrayed.

Trust will be even more difficult to develop when members are involuntary, had abusive experiences, fear that what they say can and will be used against them, have suffered numerous betrayals, or when they perceive other members as projecting aggression, and sadism. The leader who has done pre-screening and pre-assessment may know some of their social history, but other events may not be mentioned or be buried so deep that even that member remains unaware of their existence. The omitted and buried ones may be especially important in determining their ability to trust.

These, and other circumstances, can contribute to difficulty in establishing trust. From the very moment the group leader meets group members, they are assessing the leader's trustworthiness and, as the vast majority of communication is nonverbal behavior, much of the assessment and judgment is based on what and who the leader appears to be. Group leaders build trust with their understanding and acceptance that trust takes time to develop, have a willingness to accept members as they present themselves, and are able to convey caring and positive regard, faith in the group process, and empathic responding can be facilitative. These are the inner self characteristics that contribute to building trust.

Examples of Therapeutic Ruptures

Many of the events that can lead to a rupture in the therapy are likely to occur in member-to-member interactions. However, Rutan and Stone (2001) report that these tend to occur when the leader makes a mistake. Examples include when the leader either commits an insensitivity about culture and/or diversity such as a microaggression, or the leader fails to recognize and intervene when such insensitivities emerge in the session. Other leader omissions or actions that can lead to ruptures are failing to ensure equity and inclusion, forgetting important information about a group member, the timing of interventions being either too early or too late, the leader's unconscious subjective countertransference and/or failure to maintain physical, psychological, or relational boundaries.

Group leaders who recognize that they made a mistake may first want to apologize. While an apology can be forthcoming and even appropriate that may not be the best intervention therapeutically or relationally. Most people who extend an apology are sincerely trying to atone for their action or comment that was offensive or hurtful to another person. The apology is a recognition that their actions, or inactions, or comments have negatively impacted another person and may have been unintended in the sense that the actions or comment did not have a conscious intent to hurt or offend. An apology is provided with an expectation that the affected person will understand that the intent was not malicious, and that the offender wants their understanding and forgiveness. The hope and expectation are that the apology will be accepted without any effect on the relationship or on the perceptions of the offender. However, that is not all of what is transpiring, or even the most important part. Let's take a look at the real needs and impact for the group leader and for the receiver.

Assume that you are the group leader, and you offer an apology. The apology is usually offered to keep from feeling guilty or ashamed. As the leader, you may be disappointed in yourself, consider yourself as a good person with good intentions and are seeking forgiveness and the other person's approval and understanding. (While these are stated in personal terms, the same things apply to others when they extend apologies, especially between group members.)

The receiver is offended, hurt, and may even be narcissistically wounded. They may not be emotionally able to accept an apology and may feel pressured to accept the apology whether they want to or not because of social convention. For example, the receiver would be perceived as being ungracious if they were to refuse to accept the apology. The result is that the receiver is now being asked to carry their hurt and to relieve the guilt of the offender. A lose–lose situation.

Why Apologies Do Not or May Not Work

Many apologies do not work because the offender does not recognize that the offense was a narcissistic injury where the receiver had a wound to their essential self, and that this is not a minor or trivial hurt. Also, the offender usually fails to understand why what was said or done was offensive. Alternatively, they may characterize the receiver as being too sensitive, overreacting, illogical, unable to take a joke, or as lacking a sense of humor. Some offenders, such as those we see on the news or television, will say something like, "If I offended you", which is really dismissive of the receiver.

Offenders may then try to insist that they had no intention of offending and that having the receiver say or indicate that they object or are offended will often elicit the response from the offender that they are hurt that the receiver was offended. Now, the receiver has been wounded and is being charged with offending the offender. Some offenders will bring others into the discussion or solicit their support that the receiver should not be offended, or that there was nothing done that should be considered as offensive. Some will even say things such as:

- The receiver should have known that the offender meant no harm.
- The receiver ought to be able to shrug it off.
- What was said or done wasn't deliberately offensive.
- The receiver ought not to be so sensitive or quick to take offense.

All of which puts the burden on the receiver and that the receiver was wrong to be offended. Many offenders want or insist that their apology be accepted so that they will feel better.

Suggestions for How to Effectively Atone for Insensitivity and/or Microaggression

Effective atonement for an insensitivity or microaggression does not begin with an apology. It is more effective to begin with an acknowledgment of the offense and its impact on the receiver. Absent are words to indicate unintentionality, the offender's guilty feelings or an attack on the receiver, or blaming the receiver for how they or the offender feel. Acknowledgment of the offense and impact uses words to specifically state that what was said or done was hurtful, or offensive, or insensitive, or a failure to be empathic. The offender does not attempt to get away from the uncomfortable situation, or offload blame for what the receiver is feeling, or other such actions or words. After the acknowledgement described above is the time to say something like, "I'm sorry that what I did or said was hurtful or offensive or insensitive." It is best to not say something like, "I'm sorry you were hurt", which seems to convey the intention that the person should not have had the reaction that they did. Making excuses, such as "I was only trying to be funny", are also not helpful. Acknowledging, empathizing, or reflecting the receiver's feelings, and then offering an apology, is effective and usually works.

Self-absorption – Leader and Members

Self-absorption is a term that needs to be put in context, and one way of understanding what it is, how it is exhibited, and the impact it has on others is to consider it as underdeveloped and/or destructive narcissism. *Destructive narcissism pattern* (DNP) is a part of everyone's psychological development, can be age-appropriate for children and adolescents, is not pathological unless it meets the DSM diagnostic criteria, but can still be troubling to relationships, and applies to both the group leader and group members. Undeveloped and destructive narcissism are defined as unconscious and/or nonconscious attitudes and behaviors displayed by group leaders and/or members that can be very detrimental and even harmful to others. Displayed by the group leader, it can be especially harmful to some group members, such as those that are emotionally fragile, those who have insufficient psychological boundary strength and are unable to repel projections or keep from catching other people's feelings, members who are dependent and scared seeking sure answers, or those some have low self-esteem. When these behaviors and attitudes are displayed by group members, detrimental effects can be experienced both within the group for other members and the leader as well as that person's interactions and relationships with others outside of the group. Another key understanding is that either the leader or group member exhibiting the DNP behavior or attitude is unaware of their undeveloped or destructive narcissism, or of the impact it may be having on one or even all group members. There is usually no conscious intent to harm, but that does not lessen the negative effects.

Before going any further, let's define some terms, and think of narcissism as a human characteristic that is capable of being developed so that it is helpful rather than harmful, and that it is developed along a continuum reflective of age and stage of development that applies to the group leader and to the group members. References that can be helpful and provide more information include those from Kohut (1977), Brown (1998), Horwitz (2000), and Kernberg (1990).

Age-appropriate narcissism refers to expected levels of attitudes and behaviors based on chronological ages and stages of development where infants and children are expected to have considerable self-absorbed behaviors and attitudes, and adults to have few or none. *Destructive narcissism pattern* refers to adults who exhibit numerous behaviors and attitudes reflective of those expected at an earlier stage of chronological development, such as an adult who has numerous behaviors and attitudes expected of children, and these are reflected in their troubled relationships. *Narcissistic personality disorder (NPD) or pathological narcissism* behaviors and attitudes are described in the DSM-V-TR for adults (American Psychiatric Association, 2022). This description includes characteristics such as lack of empathy and an entitlement attitude. *Undeveloped narcissism* refers to having some behaviors and attitudes reflective of an earlier stage of expected development, but not as many of these, nor are they as intense or less developed than those for the Destructive Narcissistic Pattern.

Behavior and Attitude Descriptors

Let's list a few of the behaviors and attitudes that can be undeveloped or are part of a Destructive Narcissistic Pattern that may be exhibited by group leaders and group members. These are presented in three categories: the *inflated self*, *indifference to others*, and *troubling to relationships* (Brown, 2006a, 2006b).

The inflated self is categorized as grandiosity, attention-seeking, and admiration hungry. *Grandiosity* is defined as having an excessive valuation of one's and not recognizing their personal limitations. *Attention seeking* can be seen in behaviors that keeps the person as the center of attention or in the spotlight. Talking loudly, bragging, making noisy entrances and exits, frequently interrupting others, and wearing clothing that is intended to gain attention are some examples of attention-seeking behavior. *Admiration hungry* can be observed in people who actively and frequently demand or seek admiration from others. Examples include boasting, complaining, self-nominations, and looking for flattery and compliments.

Behaviors and attitudes characteristic of *Indifference to others* include extensions of self, exploitation of others and lack of empathy. *Extensions of self* is likely not in the person's awareness where they assume that others are not separate and distinct from them, that others do not have the right to be different, that others are under their control, and violations of psychological and physical boundaries are examples for this inner state that is not sufficiently separated and individuated. Other examples include giving orders and expecting to be obeyed; demanding mind reading; and entering others' space, such as an office, without knocking or waiting for an invitation. *Exploitation* is defined as manipulating others for personal gain. Examples of behaviors and attitudes include expecting favors but not returning them, and failure to recognize others' contributions, engaging in cons, scams or other ways to take advantage of others. *Lack of empathy* is exhibited when someone cannot or does not feel what other are feeling. May have the words, but not the real feelings. Examples include leaders and members who do not respond empathically, who fail to recognize and/or repair empathic failures, making insensitive comments and questions, ignoring emotionally laden disclosures and the like, and abrupt change of topic.

Troubling states reflective of undeveloped narcissism include entitlement attitudes, shallow emotions, displays of superiority, arrogance and/or contempt. *Entitlement* attitude refers to someone who has a conscious or unconscious assumption of being superior, deserving of preferential treatment, expecting deference and the like. Examples include not waiting their turn, trying to get more than their fair share, expecting others to rearrange their schedules to meet their needs, expecting to be treated as if they are unique and special by almost everyone, and frequently demanding special recognition. The person with *shallow emotions* demonstrates an inability to feel and express a wide range and variety of emotions. For example, anger can be experienced and expressed, but not annoyance and irritation. *Superiority, arrogance and contemptuous attitudes* carry the assumption that others are inferior, less worthy, and less deserving. Behavioral reflections of these attitudes include sarcasm, put-downs, demeaning and disparaging remarks, blaming, criticism, and so on.

Possible Effects on the Group and Members: Leaders

This is a very brief presentation about the possible effects of the group leader's undeveloped or destructive narcissism on the group and its members and there can be many more negative effects than are presented here. Each characteristic is presented with one example for an effect:

- *Grandiosity* – members are pushed to take dangerous psychological risks that are detrimental to their well-being.
- *Attention-seeking* – sessions become more about the leader than about the group and its members. Members' distress is overlooked or ignored.
- *Admiration-seeking* – members become more focused on ingratiation than on their concerns.
- *Extensions of self* – members can feel violated and intruded on, and that there is a lack of respect for them as individuals.
- *Exploitation* – members come to feel manipulated, taken advantage of, and not respected.
- *Lack of empathy* – members can feel diminished, devalued, or discounted and unworthy when their feelings are ignored, overlooked, or passed over.
- *Entitlement* – more time and effort is spent on getting the leader's needs met than on members' concerns, the group becomes too structured and directed.
- *Shallow emotions* – members do not receive modeling or guidance for expressing difficult and/or intense emotions.
- *Superiority* – members and the group as a whole can feel shamed, guilty, and inadequate.

Among some additional effects of the leader's self-absorption that impact the group are allowing or promoting scapegoating, not addressing boundary violations; an inability to admit to mistakes; defensiveness when challenged or a refusal to let the members express negative feelings about the leader; and failure to recognize personal limitations. Many of these can be the result of underdeveloped narcissism (Horwitz, 2000), or unresolved narcissistic needs (Gans & Alonso, 1998). Several leader attitudes and behaviors are indicative of underdeveloped narcissism (Horwitz, 2000) include but are not limited to the following:

- The inability to tolerate or accept negative criticisms or devaluation.
- Bring overly nurturing to the group or to selected group members.
- Ignoring difficult or acting out members' behavior.
- Working hard to avoid doing or saying anything that might provoke a negative response.
- Encouraging scapegoating by not intervening.
- Consciously or unconsciously seeking flattery from members.
- Responding favorably only to those members who are able to meet the leader's self-perception of being talented, having expertise, and of being very effective.

- Emotionally abusive behavior.
- Saying things and expecting them to be accepted without question.
- Refusing to admit or disclose self-doubts, uncertainty or lack of knowledge.
- Boasting about their personal lives.
- Becoming angry or hurt when a member rejects their intervention.
- The inability to be empathic.

While much of what was presented focused on the group leader, most characteristics, descriptions and effects also apply to group members. However, it is much more important that the group leader examine their behaviors and attitudes to determine if these could be contributing to some group and/or member difficulties.

Narcissistic Injury

Sensitivity to the possibility of narcissistic injury (Reich, 1972) for members is also a part of therapeutic attunement, so that these can be prevented in some instances, explored when appropriate, or used constructively to help the healing and understanding process. Narcissistic injury occurs when the essential self of the person is hurt, shamed, humiliated, or in danger of becoming destroyed. These cannot always be anticipated, nor are all of these debilitating.

Rutan and Stone (2001) perceive the group setting as a place where numerous and constant such injuries can occur as members can feel ignored, excluded, or left out, insulted, and misunderstood. For some members, the perceived slights are mild and can be overlooked or assimilated, while for others they constitute major blows to their self-esteem. Examples for group conditions and situations that may (can) result in narcissistic injury include the following:

- Frustration of dependency needs.
- Receiving no response to a disclosure, comment, question, or remark.
- The leader's decision to explore one member's issues when there are two or more competing ones. (The leader cannot win this one.)
- Emphasizing cultural and diversity differences among members instead of perceiving members as individuals.
- Empathic failures.
- Overtly or directly suggesting that a member is "wrong".
- The leader becomes distracted and "out of the group".

Reactions to narcissistic injuries are generally rage or withdrawal (Rutan & Stone, 2001; Livingston & Livingston, 1998; Kernberg, 1990). There are some narcissistic injuries that cannot be prevented because neither you nor the group members are aware of all of their sensitivities, group members do not share this personal vulnerability readily for fear that others will misuse this information, and there are individual differences for vulnerability. Stone (1992) proposes that group leaders be especially attentive to potential narcissistic injuries in the beginning stages of group where members are fearful, tentative, and less expressive or open about the little hurts. The need to be included, and a desire to not experience shame and humiliation can allow narcissistic injuries to be denied, repressed, or overlooked. Then too, the leader's need to protect his/her essential self can produce defenses that may contribute to narcissistic injury. They can be more focused on this self-protection that empathy for a member or members is not possible (Horwitz, 2000).

Stone (1992), in describing self–psychology in groups, asserts that, "Psychopathology results from narcissistic injuries" (p. 337), and that repeated or intense narcissistic injuries can produce symptoms used to restore the fragmented self. He gives Kohut and Wolfe's (1978) examples of symptoms of obsessive-compulsive behaviors, alcoholism, and chronic empty depression-like states. Stone also states that narcissistic injuries are "commonplace in everyday life" (Stone, 1992, p. 338).

It is also possible that the difficult group behaviors, and of individual members are their responses to narcissistic injury. It could be helpful for group leaders to consider this possibility whenever they think that the group, or individual members are acting out, or being difficult. The stage of group development and stage of member development play crucial roles in the decision to explore the injury in the group. When injuries are recognized and explored in the group after safety and trust are established, that process can be a valuable experience for all group members and for the leader. It is unlikely that the group or members feel safe and trusting enough for this exploration in the beginning stage. And it may be that until the second stage is navigated, where the leader is challenged and does not react defensively, and when conflicts emerge and are constructively resolved, that the group and/or members are confident that their self is not in danger of being deliberately attacked, shamed, or humiliated, that narcissistic injury can be explored and understood (Cohen, 2000). The most effective strategies for effecting identification and repair of narcissistic injury are empathy and empathic failure repair.

Repair Microaggressions and Other Insensitivities

Given the complexity and pervasiveness of cultural and diversity factors, group leaders must be aware of when a microaggression has occurred. Most of these will be microinsults or microinvalidations rather than microassaults (Sue et al. 2007). Microassaults are intentional, explicit verbal attacks such as terming someone with a demeaning label. Microinsults are rude, insensitive, and demeaning comments about a group of people and are usually unintentional but can also be intentional. Microinvalidations are unintentional but can also be intentional. Examples for microinvalidations are comments that are dismissive or devaluing of someone's experiencing of reactions to demeaning comments.

When a microaggression occurs in the group it is usually a comment is made, a question asked, or some other action that signals discrimination, bias, racism, and/or stereotyping. The incident produces the typical member and/or leader reactions such as awkwardness, uncertainty, denial on the part of the speaker and other members other than the receiver. Awkwardness results from the awareness that something offensive to someone has occurred, and social convention would dictate that it should not be acknowledged as that would not be polite and courteous. Uncertainty occurs because group members, and sometimes the group leader, are in doubt as to what to do, let it go or acknowledge it. Some members will engage in denial such as the receiver denying that they were hurt or offended, the observers can deny that they were impacted in any way, the sender or actor will deny doing anything or use the excuse that their intentions were anything but good. Some members may even deny that an incident happened. Some members who are culturally aware may have a need to be perceived as caring, unbiased, and so on, and can rush to rescue the receiver and to smooth over the incident. The experience of feeling that they are being silenced happens to both the sender and the receiver. The sender can feel silenced and blamed when the group is not accepting of the comment or other action. The receiver feels silenced when members and/or the leader do seem to understand the negative impact of the comment on them, by receiving too much comforting, not enough support or empathy, or by not receiving any empathy at all.

Possible Leader Intervention Strategy

The preliminary steps that are a part of an intervention for a microaggression are recognition of the event, observation of the impact on the sender, receiver, and other group members and, to *recognize* the incident or event as a microaggression. It is critical that the group leader *observe the impact* on the sender and on the receiver. The sender can be unaware that the incident has occurred, can feel that they are only expressing what others are thinking and feeling, and is insensitive to the impact on the receiver. The receiver can be disbelieving, narcissistically injured, and/or facing a double-bind dilemma especially when the receiver apologizes (Brown, 2019). *Observe the impact on other group members*. They too are impacted in some way and that impact may be seen in verbal and nonverbal behaviors.

The next step is for the leader to consider the *stage of group development* as that can be very important in the process for an intervention. Has sufficient trust and safety been established among the group members and with the group leader so that members will feel free to openly express their genuine thoughts, ideas, and feelings when exploring the sensitive topic. It is important that the group members not feel that they are being blamed or punished so that they become defensive and will then shut down.

If the leader decides to implement an intervention, care must be taken to be aware of the impact on the sender, the receiver and other group members throughout the process. Following is a guide for a sensitive intervention.

1   Sensitively and tactfully present the comment that was a microaggression, its impact on you as the leader, and on possible effects on relationships in the group. It is very important that neither the receiver or the sender be allowed to be treated as a joke, minimized, or dismissed as trivial or minor.
2   Empathize with both the sender and the receiver.
3   Ask the sender what message they wanted to send. Then, ask the receiver what the message was that they received.
4   Ask the receiver to state what they heard the other person say. Ask the sender to verify this or to correct any misunderstanding.
5   Ask the receiver to verbalize their feelings or reactions and the impact on them.
6   Ask the sender to first reflect what they heard said in #5 and then, to respond to that. Block apologies: the receiver should not be put in a position of taking care of the sender of the offense even if this was unintentional. It would be more helpful if the receiver were to state their reactions, Apologies can be offered later if so desired. Sometimes understanding is more affirming than an apology.
7   Ask other group members to speak openly of their reactions, thoughts, feelings, and the like.

It can be important to block apologies as these put the receiver in the double-bind position of being hurt and as also having to take care of the feelings of the person who delivered the hurt. The sender may feel peer or public pressure to accept an apology when they are not wanting to receive it or are not in a place where they can receive it. The sender can feel that they are being blamed or criticized and just want it to go away. What is important here is that the incident caused hurt whether it was intentional or not.

References

American Psychiatric Association. (2022). *Diagnostic and Statistical Manual of Mental Disorders* (5th edition). Washington, DC: American Psychiatric Association.

Aron, L. (1996). Symposium on the meaning and practice of intersubjectivity in psychoanalysis. *Psychoanalytic Dialogues*, 6, 591–597.

Ardito, R. B., & Rabellino, D. (2011, October 18). Therapeutic alliance and outcome of psychotherapy: Historical excursus, measurements, and prospects for research. *Frontiers in Psychology*, 2. Retrieved July 6, 2021, from www.frontiersin. org/articles/10.3389/fpsyg.2011.00270/.

Beebe, B., & Lachmann, F. M. (1998). Co-constructing inner and relational processes: Self- and mutual regulation in infant research and adult treatment. *Psychoanalytic Psychology*, 15(4), 480–516. doi:10.1037/0736-9735.15.4.480.

Bordin, E. S. (1979). The generalizability of the psychoanalytic concept of the working alliance. *Psychotherapy: Theory, Research & Practice*, 16, 252–260. doi:10.1037/h0085885.

Brown, N. (1998). *The Destructive Narcissistic Pattern*. Westport, CT: Praeger.

Brown, N. W. (2006a). *Coping with Infuriating, Mean, Critical People*. Westpoint, CT: Praeger.

Brown, N. W. (2006b). *Psychoeducational Groups for Non-clinical Groups Curriculum*. New York: AGPA.

Brown, N. (2019). *Conducting Effective Psychoeducational Groups*. New York: Routledge.

Cohen, B. D. (2000). Intersubjectivity and narcissism in group psychotherapy: How feedback works. *International Journal of Group Psychotherapy*. 50(2), 163–179.

Constantino, M. J., Vîslă, A., Coyne, A. E., & Boswell, J. F. (2018). A meta-analysis of the association between patients' early treatment outcome expectation and their posttreatment outcomes. *Psychotherapy*, 55(4), 473–485. doi:10.1037/pst0000169.

Elliott, R., Bohart, A. C., Watson, J. C., & Murphy, D. (2018). Therapist Empathy and Client Outcome: An Updated Meta-analysis. *Psychotherapy*, 55, 399–410.

Eubanks, C. F., Muran, J. C., & Safran, J. D. (2018). Alliance rupture repair: A meta-analysis. *Psychotherapy*, 55(4), 508–519.

Flückiger, C., Del Re, A., Wampold, B., & Horvath, A. (2018). The alliance in adult psychotherapy: A meta-analytic synthesis. *Psychotherapy*, 55(4), 316–340. doi:10.1037/pst0000172.

Gans, J. S. & Alonso, A. (1998). Difficult patients: Their construction in group therapy. *International Journal of Group Psychotherapy*, 48(3), 311–326.

Horwitz, L. (2000). Narcissistic leadership in psychotherapy groups. *International Journal of Group Psychotherapy*, 50(2), 219–235.

Kernberg, O. (1990). *Borderline Conditions and Pathological Narcissism*. Northvale, NJ: Aronson.

Kohut, H. (1977) *The Restoration of the Self*. Madison, CT: International Universities.

Kohut, H., & Wolf, E. S. (1978). The disorders of the self and their treatment: An outline. *The International Journal of Psychoanalysis*, 59(4), 413–425.

Livingston, M. & Livingston, L. L. (1998). Conflict and aggression in group psychotherapy: A self psychological vantage point. *International Journal of Group Psychotherapy*, 48, 381–391.

Norcross, J. C., & Lambert, M. J. (2018). Psychotherapy relationships that work III. *Psychotherapy*, 55(4), 303–315. doi:10.1037/pst0000193.

Reich, W. (1972). *Character Analysis*. New York: Simon & Schuster.

Rutan, S. J. & Stone, N. W. (2001). *Psychodynamic Groups Psychotherapy* (3rd ed.). New York: Guilford Press.

Stolorow, R. (1993). Thoughts on the nature and therapeutic action of psychoanalytic interpretation. In A. Goldberg (Ed.), *Progress in Self Psychology* (pp. 49–84). Hillsdale, NJ: Analytic Press.

Stone, W. N. (1992). The place of self psychology in group psychotherapy: A status Report. *International Journal of Group Psychotherapy*, 42, 335–350.

Sue, D., Capodilupo, C., Torino, G., Bucceri, J., Holder, A., Nadal, K., & Esquilin, M. (2007). Racial microaggressions in everyday life: Implications for clinical practice. *American Psychologist*, 62(4), 271–286.

Wampold, B. & Imel, Z. (2015). *The Great Psychotherapy Debate* (2nd edition). New York: Routledge.

Wright, F. (2000). The use of the self in group leadership: A relational perspective. *International Journal of Group Psychotherapy*, 50(2), 181–198.

Yalom, I. (1995). *The Theory and Practice of Group Psychotherapy*. New York: Basic Books.

8 Group Facilitation Process and Progress

Empathic Responding

There are several helpful responses for any interaction but not all of these are empathic responses. It is not suggested that the group leader is limited to only empathic responding, but it is suggested that group leaders understand why some helpful responses are not empathic. Empathic responses "perceive the internal frame of reference of another with accuracy and with the emotional components and meanings which pertain thereto as if one were the person, but without ever losing the 'as if' condition" (Rogers, 1959, pp. 210–211). Another way to phrase this is that the empathic response senses and communicates in words what the other person is feeling without losing the sense of yourself as being separate and distinct. The key words are senses and communicates what the other person is feeling. The empathy has to be conveyed to the person in words, nonverbal responses such as a facial expression are not sufficient.

Characteristics of empathic responses are being verbalized as a statement, identifying feelings and content, are kept short and focused, are non-judgmental, and accurate. It is essential that an empathic response be *verbalized* and although it can be accompanied with appropriate nonverbal gestures, that it does not rely on those gestures. Head nods, saying uh huh, leaning forward and facial expressions are not expressions of empathy.

An essential component of empathic responses is the *verbal communication of the feelings* being expressed by the person. The verbal reflection of feeling (s) uses feeling words or metaphors to show that the person's feelings were heard and understood. It is essential that this be a statement and not a question. Asking if that is what they are feeling can come after the statement. What is conveyed in a question is that the speaker is not sure of what they sensed, and it will be better to reflect what was sensed tentatively as a statement, it is not as helpful to ask it as a question. Asking if you are correct in what you sensed is acceptable if done after the statement of what was sensed. The person giving an empathic response and asking if this is correct is sending a message that they are more concerned about being correct than in responding empathically. While making an empathic

DOI: 10.4324/9781003329787-8

response can be done in concert with some nonverbal gestures such as a facial expression, it is the verbal component that is the most important part of empathic responding.

Empathic responses are *short and focused* and do not extend the person's meaning or try to interpret or ascribe possible motives or reasons for the feeling. Any additional interpretations, probing, or expansion can be done after the empathic response. For example, the empathic response has to be made before asking the person to say more about the matter.

It is important that an empathic response be *non-judgmental* and be limited to reporting what was sensed about the person's feelings. There should be no suggestion that the person's feelings were right or wrong or that they should be something other than what they were. The facial expression and voice tone of the group leader can be essential to conveying that there is no judgement about the feelings, just that these were sensed.

Accuracy of the identified feeling(s) is (are) important for the response to be empathic. The person may lack awareness that some feelings were embedded in what they said, but when these are communicated to them, they can readily agree that those embedded feelings were a part of what they were experiencing. If the attempted empathic response is not accurate, the person will usually provide a correction. Usually the correction is about the intensity of the feeling such as using the word anger, and the person feels that their experiencing was something milder like irritation, or even more intense like furious.

Helpful But Not Empathic Responses

What are some common responses that can be helpful but are not empathic (Neukrug & Schwitzer, 2006)? Nine examples of non-empathic responses that are commonly used are sympathy, paraphrasing, affirming, encouraging, questions, self-disclosure, advice, judgments and interpretations, and apologies. *Sympathy* is often conveyed to try and let the person know that someone is sorry for them and that they care. However, being sorry for someone is not the equivalent of sensing what that person is feeling and communicating this to them. *Paraphrasing* is repeating what the person said using somewhat different words and is usually focused on content. While paraphrasing is helpful to ensure that what was heard was what the speaker meant to communicate, this does not convey any sense of what the other person is or was feeling.

Affirming responses are those that reinforce the person's perspective and agreeing with that perspective. Affirming can also be a way to agree that you see them as they see themselves but does not convey any sense of what the person may be feeling.

Encouraging responses are intended to support the person and to try and give them reinforcement for what they are saying, doing or their intentions. These also are not empathic responses as they do not acknowledge what that person may be feeling.

Questions are used by many as a means to show interest in what the person is saying, to clarify, or even to suggest actions. Questions ask for more details with the thought behind these that this shows interest in the person. Some questions are asked to clarify something that may not be understood and to give the speaker an opportunity to ensure that what was heard was what they meant to say. Rhetorical questions are usually presented as "what if?" and can be attempts to get the person to think or act in a different way. The questioner already has the answer they want. Questions are not empathic responses. *Self-disclosure* responses are usually those that intend to show empathy through telling of their personal experiences that they think were similar. The thought is that empathy is understood because if experiences were similar then the feelings are similar and do not need to be spoken. It is true that experiences can be similar but no two are the same, neither may the feelings be the same, but since these are not spoken, the self-disclosure is not an empathic response. *Advice* can be presented as being an empathic response, but it is not. A thought that the advice giver may have is that they are conveying that they understand but have the knowledge of how to fix whatever it is. Again, advice is usually focused on content and providing information and not the person's feelings. *Judgments and interpretations* are not empathic responses although there are some people who think that their judgments and interpretations are helpful for the other person's understanding. These tend to evaluate the person's response or even feelings, and evaluations are not helpful or empathic. Interpretations also are not helpful and are usually extended with the thought that the person would benefit from a different perspective. Both are focused on content and not the feelings. *Apologies* are usually extended as an acknowledgement that what was done or said produced distress or injury without intent. Apologies ask the receiver for forgiveness for the act. However, apologies are not empathic responses as apologies emphasize the speaker's intent and do not acknowledge the impact on the receiver or recognize the receiver's feelings.

Empathic Failures

Kohut (1977) emphasized the importance of recognizing and repairing empathic failures and addressed here is how that can be even more critical for group therapy as the potential for their occurrence increases significantly because of the number of participants. These empathic failures also provide opportunities for therapeutic ruptures (Zilcha-Mano, 2021), narcissistic injury (Stone, 2017) and, when repaired can facilitate building the therapeutic alliance (Harris & Panozzo, 2019), facilitating a corrective emotional experience (Brown, 2021), and contributes to building group cohesion (Burlingame et al. 2018).

It is easy to have empathic failures in the group as the group leader is trying to attend to the group as a whole and its dynamics, and to individual group members in addition to monitoring their own countertransference. Just as with the nurturer in object-relations theory, it is impossible to fully anticipate the constant needs of the group and of the members and is a contributor to these failures. In addition, it is impossible to be fully empathic with everyone all of the time. The group leader has to be content with being good enough to respond empathically with some members some of the time, and to use group process commentary to respond empathically to the group as a whole when needed. However, there are some leader actions or inactions that contribute to empathic failures; the extent of their emotional presence, considering comments, remarks, or disclosures as trivial or not on topic, asking for details, not directly responding, and thinking about how to respond.

Emotional Presence

The *emotional presence* of the group leader is essential in numerous ways including to know when and how to intervene, to identify and prevent empathic failures, and/or to repair these when they occur. Leaders like group members will at times not be fully emotionally present in the session. They can become bored, think about personal concerns, find that they are thinking about there and then topics, defending against triggered feelings, composing their response and other such actions/inactions. Much can be missed when the leader is not emotionally present in the session, especially when there are emotionally laden topics that are being expressed with little affect or intensity, the topic seems surface or trivial but carry important information for the person or for the group, or when what is talked about is affecting a group member who is not expressing this except in their nonverbal behavior.

Trivializing Disclosures

Considering the input or disclosure to be trivial, or surface, or as not being important is a common way to commit an empathic failure as there can be something important embedded in what the person is saying and is not clear at that point. It is certainly possible that there is nothing significant underlying what is being said, but it could be that the person is not aware of what is lurking or embedded that is important to them. For example, in a student T-group they may be discussing schedules of courses for the next semester and embedded in that discussion could be a fear of the future that is not being directly expressed.

Asking for details can be an empathic failure because this asks the speaker to provide more content instead of first responding to their feelings. Details are seldom helpful to understand how the person feels about the situation, does not allow the person to explore their feelings, can initiate story-telling because every situation is complex with many components, and has the possibility of diluting the impact and intensity of what is being felt or experienced. Asking for details also takes it away from the here and now.

Indirect Responses

It can be very helpful for the group leader to *directly respond* to what was said and to highlight the feelings expressed or not expressed. Those feelings carry the majority of the communication's message for that person. It is not as relevant at this point to get more context, to decide if the person is overly or under responsive, to move them from the affective to the cognitive unless the intensity of their feelings seem to overwhelm them, to teach or disseminate information, ask for more details, or provide solutions. It is much more important to provide an empathic response that shows understanding and validation.

Mentally Composing a Response

Some group leaders will not be emotionally present at times because they are mentally *composing their response* to the group member. They are thinking about what they want to say instead of listening for the overt and indirect feelings about what is being expressed. Thus, much that may be important can be missed because of this inattention. Staying with the person as they are talking can allow the leader to enter the world or experiencing of the speaker and to sense what they are feeling that they may not be aware of or may be repressing or denying. Mentally composing a response is thinking about the future which prevents being fully present in the here and now.

Other common behaviors for leaders and members that contribute to empathic failures are changing the topic or subject, wanting to flee, wanting to or asking questions, labeling the behavior or inferring motives, and ignoring emotionally remarks or disclosures. It can be uncomfortable to be fully present with some disclosures, but that can increase the possibility of empathic failures.

Eliminate Empathic Failures

Group leaders will find that reducing and/or eliminating empathic failures will enhance the group process, promote trust and safety and encourage members in deeper self-reflection and exploration. Among the many benefits are the following.

- Strengthens the therapeutic relationship. Empathic responding sets up a link that allows the receiver to feel heard, understood and validated. This link can play a major role in the members' willingness to self-disclose, to feel connected to the group and to the leader, and can allow them to perceive the leader and group as calming and safe where they will be valued and supported which build trust.

- Models effective communication skills. When the leader repairs empathic failures this demonstrates good communication skills, and the value of responding to the speaker's feelings as well as the content. Communications in the group and in members' relationships can be more effective when attention is given to recognizing when there may have been an empathic failure which helps teach members better relating and communication skills.

- Taps into the metacommunication of the message. Repairing empathic failures illustrates that the metacommunication was the most important part of the message, that the feelings expressed or unexpressed were the most significant component of the message, and that although it was belated, that the speaker's message was heard and understood.

- Repairs and prevents ruptures of the therapeutic alliance. Empathic failures can cause ruptures in the therapeutic alliance with the leader as the leader can be perceived in idealizing terms, someone who is all knowing and all powerful. Further, the failure does not recognize and reflect the speaker's self-perception as being worthwhile and valid. Ruptures can easily occur when someone feels minimized, ignored, dismissed, avoided and the like which is all too likely with empathic failures.

- Can provide a corrective emotional experience. It could be that some members have experienced empathic failures frequently where their feelings were not recognized and responded to, they were admonished to not feel the way that they do or were simply ignored. Initiating a repair in the group could begin a healing process. Repairing a failure in the group could be the first, or only, or one of the few times that their feelings were given the attention that these merited.

- Reassures group members that they are heard and understood. When a failure is repaired it not only addresses that particular member but also reassures other group members that they will be attended to, heard, and understood. The process of the repair also models how such repairs can be done and members can then learn to use this in other relationships.

- Helps to heal narcissistic injuries. Narcissistic injuries are wounds to the essential self (Cohen, 2000; Kohut & Wolfe, 1978; Stone, 2017) that have the potential to produce narcissistic rage. While narcissistic injuries are encountered across the life span, these are seldom healed and negatively affect the person's self-esteem and even their relationships with others. Repairing empathic failures in the group setting can help start a process for healing these long-term and enduring injuries.

Group-Level Empathic Failures

The group leader also has a responsibility to stay in touch with the group as a whole entity and to work to identify and repair empathic failures that occur at the group level. Some examples for group-level empathic failures include the following.

- Forgetting important details about members' disclosures especially those that have commonalties.
- Not realizing the impact of a disclosure on the group as a whole. Empathic failure repair usually focuses on the individual group member that was empathically failed and much too often the impact on the remainder of the group is not addressed which provides the empathic failure for the group as a whole. Empathic failures can also have an impact on the group's perception of trust and safety, resistance and willingness to disclose.
- When the leader forgets major discussions, topics, disclosures and the like from previous sessions. So much can happen in sessions that it can be understandable that the leader may not remember some of what took place in some sessions. This is why it is essential that the group leader make some notes immediately after sessions that include the major topics and other material that emerged during the session and to read these before beginning the next session. The leader's forgetting can signal to the members a level of disinterest, reduced caring and concern, and/or as being of little or no importance.
- Ignoring conflicts and their impact on the group. Conflicts can be expected in group and can range from mild disagreements and differences of opinion or perception to intense and important clashes. Some group leaders have such a low tolerance for conflict at any level until they work to suppress it and that can lead to ignoring them for the leader's comfort. That affects the group and is a message to group members that conflict is not tolerated. In addition, if or when conflicts emerge whether managed or resolved, and the leader does not recognize or address the impact of the conflict on the group, that becomes a group-level empathic failure. It is important to not only work with the individual group members in the conflict, it is also essential to address the impact of that conflict on other group members, and at times on the group entity.
- Underestimating or minimizing the leader's absence from a session, or their illness that reduces their ability to be emotionally present. The leader's physical and emotional presence makes a difference to the group so that when they are absent even with good reason, the group feels that absence and it can be important for the leader to give members an opportunity to express how that absence affected them.
- Failure to recognize and repair the group's as well as individual group members' narcissistic injuries from microaggressions. This is a huge empathic failure and it is very important that group leaders recognize microaggressions, stay fully aware of the possible narcissistic injuries that may occur and work to repair these as soon as possible.

- Failure to recognize shame. This can be another huge empathic failure that is very wounding to the person. Indeed, some group members may choose to leave the group if they are shamed or witness another member being shamed. While the leader may not be the one that triggers that shame, it is the leader's responsibility to recognize and repair that empathic failure.
- Not enforcing rules and boundaries. Rules and boundaries are instituted to provide safety and trust for group members so when the group leader fails to enforce these, that can produce some uncertainty and lack of trust that they will be adequately taken care of. Reducing uncertainty and ambiguity is important for the functioning of the group and to help produce group cohesion. Group members are also looking for equitable treatment which does not happen when rules and/or boundaries are violated and there is no consequence for doing so.
- Failure to adequately monitor countertransference. This is another huge reason for empathic failures and one that can easily occur as the countertransference is likely to be unconscious on the leader's part. Many decisions about what to respond to or not respond, to probe, to encourage can be influenced by the leader's unconscious countertransference and it is wise for the leader to try and monitor this.

Empathic Failure Repair Procedures

The first step is to recognize that the person did not receive a response, received an inappropriate response such as a question, or only the content was responded to but not the feelings or any number of other responses that were not empathic.

Once the failure is recognized, use one of the following four guides.

- Say to the person, "I did not respond when you were expressing (name the feeling(s) the person was expressing or trying to express), and I want you to know that I did hear and understand. It would have been more helpful if I could have told you that I heard you at that time."
- If you tuned out and did not hear what they said, or only a part of it say something like the following. "I did not hear or respond to you when you were trying to express something important to you. That was not helpful." Saying what you did hear and understand could be added, if it did not emphasize that you were not listening.
- If you responded inappropriately, e.g. advice, you could say the following. "When you were talking about _____ I (whatever the inappropriate response was) instead of letting you know that I heard and understood that you were _____ (feelings expressed by the person). If I had let you know I did hear your feelings it may have been more helpful than (whatever you did)."

- If you failed to report on triggered personal feelings you could say something like the following. "When you were expressing your feelings about _____, I did not let you know that I was feeling _____. I realize that knowing how you affected me could have been useful to you."

This script is intended to give leaders a guide for how to start repairing an empathic failure. It is important that leaders develop their own unique script for these times.

Cultural Determinants and Group Culture

Culture is both macro and micro: macro in the sense of the larger environment such as the community, city or country; and micro in the sense of family or social group. These culturally determined conventions, rules, and norms to be mandates that guide the person's understanding of acceptable and unacceptable behavior. These culturally determined norms influence group members to think, act and feel in concert with what they have internalized as appropriate norms (Forsyth, 1999). Further, these also determine what can and cannot be talked about and with whom and is complex and mostly a hidden norm. These hidden cultural determinants can make therapy difficult as the group leader is asking group members to go against some ingrained understandings and behaviors attitude that were reinforced since birth. This discussion refers to culturally determined norms for the individual group member as social convention.

Building a group culture where members are able to accept open, honest and direct communication, and process commentary is critical to the group's movement through stages of development as well as fostering the psychological growth and development for members. Agazarian (1997), and Yalom (1995) provide some specific information to guide the group leader in developing a group's culture that facilitates communication among members to promote interpersonal learning, and acceptance of group process commentary. Presented here are cultural determinants and group culture, social convention as a barrier, social convention defenses and group communication patterns, leader social defenses, and effects of social convention and defenses on group process commentary.

Social Convention as a Barrier

Major barriers to developing are the social conventions that members acculturated from their culture that can prevent establishing the desired group culture and that have an impact on process commentary. The impacts of social conventions begin at birth and continue throughout life, and some are specifically taught while others are unconsciously introjected, internalized, and become a part of the self. The unconscious and non-conscious conventions, norms, and taboos that were taught and internalized are influential and acted on without conscious awareness.

Reflection or discussion questions: Were there topics or events that were not supposed to be disclosed outside of the immediate family? How does or would that impact or influence your communications in the group?

Social Convention Defenses

Social defenses are employed to prevent violations of culturally determined social conventions. These defenses can be categorized as cognitive, somatic, masochistic, and sadistic (Agazarian, 1997). These defenses in the group help members to avoid authenticity, deflect them from the real task, establish their status in the group, define the rules of relationships among and between members, and maintain boundaries.

Social defenses are employed to keep the real Self from being seen by others for fear of rejection, destruction, or other fantasized negative consequences, such as, "Others won't like me", "They'll ignore or avoid me", "They may hurt me". *Deflecting* from the real task allows members to avoid intimacy, preserve their false persona, suppress important feelings, keep the group from being present-centered, and to refrain from self-exploration and self-reflection. Common strategies for deflecting include intellectualizing, talking about feelings instead of expressing feelings, introducing there and then topics, giving advice, and acting as an identified patient. The status members have in the group determines, in part, the extent to which they are included or excluded, the deference expected and/or received, the affection attracted and the quality of acceptance and approval received from other members. The rules of relationship or engagement are messages sent and received by group members about the degree of intimacy that is desired, or that can be tolerated, a willingness to let oneself be known, appropriate and acceptable personal topics for verbalizing, and if input from others will be valued. Psychological boundaries allow protections for the self from the potential threats in the everyday world. Those people without sufficient boundaries, or boundary strength, run risks of becoming enmeshed, overwhelmed or destroyed by others who unconsciously, have needs of power and control, underdeveloped narcissism, or other unresolved issues that do not recognize the rights of others.

The two main ways that social defenses are used in the group are social talk, and social flights (Agazarian, 1997). Social talk allows the group member to appear friendly without being a friend, and that conveys no personal or factual information. The other manifestation is social flight which can be observed actions such as answering a question with a question, changing the subject of the conversation, interrupting a speaker, discounting what a member says, insinuations or speculations, sarcasm, gossip, funny stories and victimizing jokes, monologues, and "know it all" pontification.

Discussion: What are some ways that social talk could be manifested in a group session, such as traffic, holidays, team sports, television, and the like?

Social Defenses and Group Communication Patterns

Observing communication patterns in group sessions reveals what social defenses are used. Agazarian (1997) describes six communication patterns that members can use:

- "As if" statements.
- Emotional inferiority.
- Emotional superiority.
- Intellectual superiority.
- Moral righteousness.
- Self-protection.

"As if" statements are made to sound like the person is involved, but in reality, these statements are used to keep the speaker safe and protected. These are yes–but responses that start out as agreeing and end on the other side. These communications are ambiguous and full of redundancies. Examples of "as if" statements are:

- "I don't know what you want."
- "I want to do what you suggest, but ___."

The first statement implies that the person would do what is wanted if only it was clear what was wanted. In actuality what the person is saying is that, as long as they can claim confusion, they do not have to act or to become involved. The second statement is a disguised way of saying that the speaker has no intention of doing what was suggested, but does not want to run the risk of offending, or of appearing uncooperative by saying so openly.

Emotional inferiority occurs when the speaker assumes an inferior stance compared to others. Putting oneself down and discounting one's self in direct or hidden ways reflects this defense. Some behaviors that reflect emotional inferiority are complaining, becoming more needy, expecting others to read your mind, and being the scapegoat or identified patient. There always seems to be someone in the group who rushes to take care of this person either for self-soothing reasons, or because that is their characteristic behavior. All involved are using social defenses to maintain distance and superficiality.

Emotional superiority can be seen as a characteristic of grandiosity but may be the defense to hide their fears and feelings of inferiority. They boast and brag about accomplishments, belongings, people they associate with, and are overly confident about their abilities. They are unwilling to listen to others, will frequently interrupt and correct others including the leader, and can become irritated when their superiority is not acknowledged.

Intellectual superiority seeks to use social expectations to exert power and influence without openly seeming to do so. This social defense put others on the defensive and allows the focus to be shifted to the cognitive, the impersonal or, to the person put on the defensive. The communication pattern for this defense is exhibited by:

- challenges,
- persuasion,
- argument,
- interruptions,
- interpretations,
- giving advice, and/or
- asking leading questions.

In all these instances, the speaker not only avoids revealing any personal information or feelings, they maintain a spotlight on other topics or people.

Moral righteousness is not taking a stand or supporting personal moral and ethical values. That would be honest and genuine. Moral righteousness is a finger pointing blaming stance that is intended to produce shame and guilt in the other person, and to shore up personal feelings of superiority. "I'm better than you are." is the theme of the moral righteousness social defense communication pattern. Verbal interactions will contain words, such as should, ought, always and never, applied to the other person(s). This communication can tap wishes, fears, old parental messages, and the deep-seated fear that the self is not good enough and may be fatally flawed.

Self-protection may be the defense for some who can keep the attention and interest in the group with funny stories, jokes, gossip, and so on. They always seem to know how to keep the session flowing, and their social skills can make them the life of the party. However, this behavior also functions to protect the person from intimacy, and from their real self being revealed. As long as the conversation is on another topic or person, they are satisfied. The interest and excitement engendered by telling jokes, and so on, are icing on the cake. They will now be sought out and perceived as someone who has something interesting and/or funny to say. You never get to see the real person behind the smokescreen.

Reflection: Identify which of the above social defenses you use most frequently when interacting with others or in a group. How do you think this defense would impact the interpersonal relationships in the group?

Leaders' Social Defenses

Leaders too can mount social defenses. The most common leader defense is termed one up - one down by Agazarian (1997). This defense can be observed in behaviors such as dissonance between what is said and what is done, avoiding contact by not emotionally connecting with members, and sending double bind messages. The leader uses the position to maintain power, control and anonymity.

The status defense is extremely difficult to avoid as both the leader and group members' use it, although for different reasons. Members arrive at the group expecting the leader to be an authority and to take care of them. Indeed, the leader has to fulfill both functions to some extent. These functions become a defense when members continue their dependency over a period of time, refuse to accept responsibility for their own treatment, and are very threatened by the leader's attempts to promote separation and individuation. Leaders use the defense to maintain power, control, and to meet personal dependency needs. The leader who does not empower members to take responsibility for their treatment and progress, encourages dependency, wants to be the expert, and to make brilliant interpretations and interventions, is using the status defense.

Effect on Group Process Commentary

Yalom (1995) describes three social convention taboos that can affect how group process commentary is received: observation, comments, and lack of challenges to the leader. Understanding these social convention taboos are helpful to the group leader as preparation for making group process commentary to better understand members' reactions when commentary is provided. These taboos seem to apply for most or many cultures. The observation taboo is to not closely monitor or stare at another person as this can be perceived as rude, threatening, forcing intimacy and is uncomfortable for that person. Another taboo identified by Yalom (1995) is to not comment on others observed behavior as this can be perceived by the person as they are doing something shameful or wrong. The final taboo is to not allow reciprocal process observation and commentary which means that members are not supposed to challenge the group leader as this can evoke anxieties around parents and other authority figures.

Teaching group members to accept process commentary is a critical task for the group leader. However, members generally are not ready for or knowledgeable about it and must be gently and sensitively led to doing and accepting something that turns their conventional ways of behaving and thinking upside down.

Group Co-leaders

There are numerous configurations for co-leaders. Co-leaders can be colleagues, trainees and supervisors, couples, as examples. While there are positives for having a co-leader

Yalom and Leszcz (2021) state that "You are far better off leading a solo group with good supervision than being locked into an incompatible co-therapy relationship." Discussed are the positives for having co-leaders, the disadvantages, and how to form a mutually satisfying co-leader relationship.

Advantages and Disadvantages

Positive advantages include not having to assume full responsibility for the group and its functioning, receiving encouragement and support, it becomes possible to identify and repair empathic failures more readily, and can enrich the group experience for group members. Assuming that the co-leaders are compatible with each other, it is comforting to be able to rely on the other person to assume some of the responsibility for how the group functions and develops, and not have sole responsibility for this. Co-leaders can encourage and support each other as well as identifying helpful actions and interventions such as group process commentary. Co-leading can lessen the responsibility for the individual group leader to identify and repair empathic failures as one of them is always acting as an observer and can step in when an empathic failure is missed. In addition, by having two leaders each of which brings their unique selves to the therapy, group members and the group can be enriched by the uniqueness of each leader.

Additional advantages include having greater cognitive and observational range, may generate more hunches and strategies; flexibility for leader's attendance, mutual respect, reduces anxiety, provide feedback, and they may capitalize on each other's strengths.

Disadvantages fall into one or more of these categories: unequal roles, dual roles, evaluative component, distributes the focus for members, and can arouse suspicion among group members. Disadvantages for the co-leaders include triggering unconscious fears, monitoring countertransference, and leaders' differences for theoretical perspectives.

No matter how well intentioned, co-leadership produces unequal roles especially for the trainee/supervisor leaders. The recommended agreement established prior to the start of the group can be helpful to clarify and specify the roles each leader will assume in the group sessions. However, there are some leader characteristics that will also affect the roles to make them unequal as the group members will tend to favor one over the other. While this may be easier to detect with the trainee/supervisor, the inequality for other co-leader relationships is also present. Common unequal roles can be held around leaders' ages, race/ethnicity, professional status, gender, sexual identity, and other cultural factors depending on those of the group members.

Another constraint or disadvantage is that the co-leaders may have dual roles with each other. Examples for dual roles can be trainee/supervisor, marriage/committed relationships, relatives, or any relationships outside of the group that the co-leaders have.

The evaluative component between or among the co-leaders can affect not only the relationship but also the actions of each in the group setting. This can be especially important for the trainee/supervisor relationship but can also be present for other relationships as the evaluative component affects the well-being of the leader being evaluated as well as their having to constantly monitor their reactions and input or interventions.

It can also be that the co-leaders are not as emotionally present or group focused as would be expected or needed as their focus may be more on the relationship than on the group. This could result in failures to intervene, to identify group processes, and to identify and repair empathic failures. It is most helpful to the group and its members when the leader and co-leaders can be fully focused on the group.

Group members can be suspicious about what the co-leaders talk about among themselves outside of the group. Group members are asked to bring all discussions about the group that they have with other group members outside of the sessions back into the group so that other members know what is being said about them and/or the group. However, this is not a requirement for co-leaders and because of their professional responsibilities it may not be feasible for them to bring all of their outside discussions back into the group. It is important that co-leaders recognize that group members have concerns about their outside of the group discussion about them and to make some efforts to summarize their outside the group discussions to bring back into the group.

Tip: Co-leaders can summarize the major topics they discussed about the group and report on these to the group. Major topics such as theme for the session, major topics for the session and possible co-leader empathic failures.

Disadvantages for the co-leaders can be that their unconscious fears about their group leadership adequacy are triggered which can be especially important for the trainee/supervisor co-leaders. Co-leaders may find it more difficult to monitor their countertransference as their attention is dispersed on the group and its members as well as on the other co-leader. It can be more difficult to identify their reactions as stemming from their personal issues, the relationship with the other co-leader or from the group and its members.

One of the most difficult differences to address among the co-leaders is when they have differing theoretical perspectives which can lead to ruptures for their relationship and have an unconscious effect on the group. There may even be differences among them when they both seem to have the same theoretical perspective but may vary that in some way.

The primary disadvantage/ dissatisfaction flows from the problems in the relationship between the two co-therapists such as when they have differing theoretical perspectives, conscious or unconscious competition needs or when they have different professional languages.

Agreements

Yalom and Leszcz (2021) and others recommend that the co-leaders have an agreement among them that is worked out prior to the start of the group. It may not be necessary to have a written agreement, but in some cases it could be helpful. The agreement would address the following:

- Interventions and speaking time to specify how it will be determined which co-leader provides an intervention, if they switch off and alternate, or another option and how they want to determine speaking time so that one co-leader is not seen as dominating.

  −Tip: One alternative is that they agree that when an intervention is provided that co-leader finishes the intervention before the other co-leader interjects.

- How conflicts among the co-leaders will be managed.

  −Tip: Plan to resolve conflicts/disagreements outside of the group session not in the group as these conflicts tend to be primarily about the relationship.

- Deciding how they want to manage the group, such as who leads off, if they invite the other to contribute, who summarizes, when and how process illumination takes place and other tactics that will promote the group's and members' growth and development.

  - *Tip: Co-leaders should avoid having both leaders do everything or anything. That can be confusing for group members. Some effective strategies are to either have one be the leader for all sessions, or to switch leaders each session, or to have one be lead for three to four sessions. The deciding factor is to not have seemingly competition among leaders or to be confusing for group members.*

- Consultation and planning.

  −Tip: It is helpful for co-leaders to consult before and after the group session so as to organize and plan the session and to touch base before the session begins especially if there needs to be changes for what was planned.

- Managing glitches, possible therapeutic ruptures, and the like.

  −Tip: Agree on how to intercede when one leader does not notice, is ignoring, avoiding, or going in an unproductive direction. It's best to work this out prior to the start of the group and will prevent leader's being in conflict during a session.

- Organize and manage group tasks.

  −Tip: Decide if there will be a summary of the session at the end of the session or at the beginning of the next session and which co-leader provides that. One variation for co-leading is that one is the active leader, and the other is the process observer. When this is used, then the process observer will be expected to do the summarizing and reporting.

No matter how well intentioned and how hard they try one co-leader will be most dominant. A recommended way to manage this is to first recognize that it is happening and for the co-leaders to discuss this among themselves, not in the group and not with the group. This is a relationship matter that should be worked out among them.

References

Agazarian, Y. (1997). *Systems-Centered Therapy for Groups*. New York: Guilford Press.

Brown, N. (2014). *Facilitating Challenging Groups*. New York: Taylor & Francis.

Brown, N. (2021). The significance and importance of repairing empathic failures. In Y. I. Kane, S. Masselink, & A. Weiss (Eds.), *Women, Intersectionality and Power in Group Psychotherapy*. New York: Routledge.

Burlingame, G. M., McClendon, D. T., & Yang, C. (2018). Cohesion in group therapy: A meta-analysis. *Psychotherapy*, 55(4), 384–398. doi:10.1037/pst0000173.

Cohen, B. D. (2000). Intersubjectivity and narcissism in group psychotherapy: How feedback works. *International Journal of Group Psychotherapy*. 50(2), 163–179.

Dugo, J. & Beck, A. (1997). Significance and complexity of early phases in the development of the co-therapy relationship. *Group Dynamics: Theory, Research and Practice* 1, 284–305.

Forsyth, D. (1999). *Group Dynamics* (3rd ed.) Pacific Grove, CA: Brooks/Cole.

Freedman, W. & Diedrich, L. (2017). Group co-facilitation: creating a collaborative partnership. In M. Ribeiro, J. Gross, & M. Turner (Eds.), *The College Counselor's Guide to Group Psychotherapy*. New York: Routledge.

Harris, B. A. & Panozzo, G. (2019). Therapeutic alliance, relationship building, and communication strategies-for the schizophrenia population: An integrative review. *Archives of Psychiatric Nursing*, 33(1), 104–111. doi:10.1016/j.apnu.2018.08.003.

Kohut, H. (1977). *The Restoration of the Self*. Madison, CT: International Universities.

Kohut, H., & Wolf, E. S. (1978). The disorders of the self and their treatment: An outline. *The International Journal of Psychoanalysis*, 59(4), 413–425.

Luck, M. & Hackney, H. (2007). Group coleadership: A critical review. *Counselor Education and Supervision* 46, 280–293.

Neukrug, E & Schwitzer, A. (2006). *Skills and Tools for Today's Counselors and Psychotherapists*. Pacific Grove, CA: Brooks/Cole.

Rogers, C. (1959). *Client-Centered Therapy*. Boston, MA: Houghton Mifflin.

Roller, B. & Nelson, V. (1991). *The Art of Co-therapy: How Therapists Work Together*. New York: Guilford Press.

Stone, W. (2017). Self-psychology: Empathy and process. *International Journal of Group Psychotherapy*, 67(1), 164–170.

Yalom, I. (1995). *The Theory and Practice of Group Psychotherapy*. New York: Basic Books.

Yalom, I. & Leszcz, M. (2021). *The Theory and Practice of Group Psychotherapy* (6th edition). New York: Basic Books.

Zilcha-Mano, S. (2021). Toward personalized psychotherapy: The importance of the trait-like/state-like distinction for understanding therapeutic change. *American Psychologist*, 76(3), 516–528. doi:10.1037/amp0000629.

9 Managing Group Difficulties

Group leaders will encounter some difficult situations in their groups and what is discussed here are some common difficulties and how these may be managed for the benefit of the group and members. Difficulties have to be sensitively managed as they affect both the particular group member and the group as a whole as members will expect that they will be treated the same way as the difficult member. While it is not possible to foresee or prevent some of the difficult situations, such as conflict which is almost always present in a group, it is possible to use them in a constructive way to promote healing, growth, and insight.

Narcissistic Injury

Narcissistic injury occurs when the essential self of the person is hurt, shamed, humiliated, or in danger of becoming destroyed (Reich, 1972). These cannot always be anticipated, nor are all of these debilitating. The leader's sensitivity to the possibility of narcissistic injury for members is also a part of therapeutic attunement, so that these can be prevented in some instances, explored when appropriate, or used constructively to help the healing and understanding process.

Some negative impacts for members encountering narcissistic injury and on the progress of the group were described in Chapter 7. These impacts are not usually overt and visible which is one reason why they may go undetected and exert their negative influences without the leader's or other members' conscious awareness. Group leaders are encouraged to consider the possibility of potential narcissistic injury for one or more group members as an explanation for their behavior or behavior change such as they become defensive, resistant, silent and/or withdrawn, attempt to deflect the discussion, attacking the leader or other group members, initiating a conflict with another group member or members, openly expressing dissatisfaction with the group and/or leader, questioning the personal value of the group for them, fomenting dissention among group member and the like.

Group leaders can also use their own internal reflection and experiencing as a guide for identifying possible narcissistic injury such as becoming

DOI: 10.4324/9781003329787-9

confused in the session, feeling misunderstood, becoming uncertain about how to proceed or intervene whereas before they were not uncertain, or having a feeling that they didn't see or understand something important and other such reflections. Reflections after the session(s) and/or consultation with a supervisor or mentor can help to clarify matters especially if there was an unrecognized narcissistic injury.

Possible interventions for narcissistic injury in the session or at a subsequent session will be empathic failure repair as noted in Chapter 7. The details of the possible injury do not need to be identified or probed, it is sufficient for the leader to note that they missed or may have missed some important feelings about the topic under discussion and to then identify what may have been missed. It is best to let the individual group member decide what to disclose or if to disclose their narcissistic injury.

Conflict

The open emergence of conflict in the group can be very threatening for some group members, and for some group leaders who have life experiences that predispose them to fear conflict because of possible unpleasant and negative outcomes. Thus, any disagreement arouses their fear and dread, and they work hard to maintain harmony, ignore the conflict, or withdraw. They have not learned or accepted the value of working through conflicts to reach constructive and acceptable solutions, or in being comfortable with a decision by all to disagree on this particular point or issue and move on without negative impact on the relationship(s). When leaders fear conflict they work hard to ensure that conflict does not emerge in the group, or they ignore conflict, suppress it, and use a wide variety of strategies to keep from having to deal with it. This seldom works because conflicts are a natural part of life, are always present in some form in every group and, when not openly acknowledged and addressed, work on a nonconscious level to negatively affect the group and individual members.

The first step for leaders is to become more comfortable with a higher level of conflict, and the second step is to identify open and disguised conflict among members. Becoming more comfortable with conflict is a part of the leader's personal development which is addressed in previous chapters. The focus here is on working with conflicts as they emerge in the group, and presentation of material that can be used with groups whose focus is on conflict resolution.

Vignette

> *The interpersonal process group that Bill was leading had met for several weeks, and although there had been some minor friction between some members, they seemed to be progressing and gaining in their interpersonal learning. The friction was not ignored when it appeared, and Bill tried to get members to work through their disagreements*

rather than to dismiss them as unimportant. *Some members were more active than others with the eldest female group member taking the lead to talk when silences fell. Other members were content with her behavior and expressed appreciation for her openness about her background and current concerns.*

About midway during the sixth session, the group became silent. Up to that point they had discussed their progress toward their personal goals for the group and seemed to feel satisfied with what they had accomplished. This silence became prolonged, and Bill began to feel anxious and tense. After several minutes of silence, he told the group that this silence felt different from other silences that had occurred in the group, and that he felt himself becoming more anxious and tense. No one responded. He invited group members to speak about their current experiences at this moment in the group, but no one said anything. Bill told the group that he was puzzled by their silence and unresponsiveness but did not push for responses. The members sat in silence for the remainder of the group.

Bill was sure that the next session would reveal the cause(s) for the silence and decided that he would not push for an explanation at this time but would explore this with the group when the time seemed right. He would let the group guide the session to fulfill their needs. The group began with Bill asking if there was any unfinished business and received no response. He asked if there were any important and urgent concerns that members were bringing to the group, but again there was no response. Bill decided to let the silence unfold as in his experience, one or more group members would become anxious enough to speak and break the silence. However, this did not happen for this group, and they remained stubbornly mute. Bill tried making a process comment, but that too received no response. He directed questions and requests for input to specific group members, and they would give short and unresponsive answers. The session felt tense and miserable to Bill, and he projected that it probably felt that was to members.

During the week between sessions, Bill met with or talked on the phone with each group member to explore with them their silence, and thoughts about the group's silence. All members said that they were satisfied with the group although they did not like the prolonged silence, did not understand the silence, and were not suppressing conflict with another member or with the leader. Bill encouraged each to speak about their feelings concerning the silence in the next session, and each member agreed to do so, but did not follow through even when Bill reminded them of their agreement. The group was stubbornly mute. Bill was at his wits end; he did not understand the group's silence, and nothing so far had worked.

Redefining personal thoughts about the nature of conflict can aid in identification. All conflicts are not battles, attacks, and the like, they are also disagreements, differences of interest, opinions and/or values, disputes, and dissensions. Conflicts range from mild to intense, and are best dealt with as they emerge. The leader and members may also need to redefine their expectations about the outcomes for conflict to move away from a win–lose perspective to a negotiating-problem solving one where each person's perspective is valued and respected, and the relationship is strengthened.

When a conflict emerges and is identified as such, leaders should listen and gauge the intensity of feelings for each participant openly expressing the disagreement, and observe the nonverbal intensity for those group members who are not actively involved at the present time. First, acknowledge the recognition of the conflict and, either ask about the intensity of feelings, or make a reflective response that identifies the intensity. It can be especially important and helpful to immediately continue to work with conflicts that have strong and intense feelings triggered. This can be more important than continuing to work on the other goals for the session. Also, leaders may want to ask other group members about their feelings and intensity as they listen to the members having a conflict.

Resolution Facilitation Strategies

There are some ground rules that can facilitate the process.

- The leader must appear to be in control and should guide and facilitate the process.
- Intervene to keep members from choosing sides.
- No name calling or demeaning comments.
- Include the whole group in the process as indicated in the following procedure.

A. Procedure for Addressing Conflict in the Group

1 Assess the emotional intensity for each person involved in the conflict. Note body positions, gestures, voice tone and quality, word choice, facial expression, and the leader's reactions.
2 Acknowledge the disagreement, differences, or conflict.
3 Ask each person to describe their feelings at the moment; could also have them rate the intensity of the feelings using the range from 0 (no intensity) to 10 (extreme intensity).
4 Ask other group members to report their feelings. These could also be rated by members using the same scale in step 3.
5 Judge whether to continue or not. If the emotional intensity is rated 3 or below, the conflict may not need addressing at this time.
6 Ask members in the conflict if they want to work through the conflict.

    a   If both say yes – continue by using the negotiation.
    b   If both say no – stop at this point.
    c   If one member says yes, and the other says no, then work with the member who says no to understand the resistance.

B. One Member Has High Emotional Intensity

After completing steps 1–6 proceed as follows.

1 Work with the member who has high emotional intensity.

a Ask him/her to define the conflict as he/she perceives it.
b Listen carefully and assess if the conflict is one of the following.

    i A clash of opinions.
    ii A clash of values.
    iii Any misunderstandings or errors of fact.
    iv A clash of interests where the member with high emotional intensity.
    v could potentially lose something of importance to him/her.

c Repeat steps a and b for the other person(s) in the conflict
d Label the conflict as (i), (ii), or (iv), and correct misunderstandings and errors if no. (iii).
e Get agreement, or not, to work on the conflict from all involved.
f Continue to work with the high intensity member(s).
g Ask them to describe what it is like to have a different perspective with the feelings they reported earlier.
h Ask them to rate the intensity of their feelings at the moment. (There can be some reduction from the previous rating. If there is no reduction, proceed on a hypothesis that there could be some transference or projection present, and be very tentative.)
i Reflect the feelings and perspective. Ask the other person if these mirror their feelings, or are they different, even when the emotional intensity was lower for them from the beginning.
j If the member's emotional intensity is still high (above 3), ask what would it take to bring it down.
k Try a short breathing exercise for self-calming, and do another check-in with the person.
l Ask if there is an association with a previous experience where he/she had similar feelings. Listen to the story and reflect content and feelings.
m Ask if there might be some residual feelings from the previous experience that may be influencing their perception of the current experience. The answer will probably be yes, but even if the member does not see the association, they will start to reflect on that possibility. Do not push for acceptance of the possible association.
n Do a check-in with the other person in the conflict, and with other group members. Reassess the high emotional intensity member's rating. It should be low enough at this point to cease this procedure. If the emotional intensity is still too high, use breathing or meditation for further calming.
o It is probably best to stop working on the conflict at this point, and initiate a discussion about the procedure. This will introduce a cognitive focus that also helps to reduce residual intensity and tension.

    p   Or, if both have reduced intensity, proceed with the negotiation process.

C. Both Participants Have High Intensity

1   Initiate steps 1–6. Work with both members, switching back and forth during the process, but pay particular attention to step 4 as other group members may have "caught" the high intensity, or because of their own past experiences. The steps described in 7a–p can be followed, again switching between members in the conflict.

When conflicts produce highly intense feelings that are linked to projections, transference, or fears; the leader can expect the issue to remain unresolved for the time being, and to re-emerge in some form in later sessions. When it does re-emerge, the intense feelings will be reduced, and the negotiation process can be used. One or more members will also have reflected on the conflict, and can help provide a more objective perspective. What is detrimental to the group will be to suppress or deny that there is still work to be done on the conflict, or that there are residual feelings that may need attention.

Conflict and Group Stage

Conflict, no matter how mild, is usually present in all groups from the beginning of the group, and the stage of group development is an important consideration in the leader's decision about managing it. Some suggested leader strategies follow for each stage.

- Stage 1: Quick intervention, sell members on expressing thoughts, feelings, and ideas; and convince them of the benefits of working through the conflict. Determine group members' dread, fear of conflict, past experiences, and need for support.
- Stage 2: Expect conflict. Encourage expression and working through conflict. Assess members' comfort levels with conflict often.
- Stage 3: Conflict is likely to be suppressed in the quest to maintain harmony. Encourage members to express and work through mild differences, and to explore their previous experiences for clues to their reactions.
- Stage 4: Conflict re-emerges because of impending termination. Leader's process to connect to termination and encourage working through.

Vignette

> *A conflict had broken out between two male members when one accused the other of being bigoted, and the accused responded that his religion was not bigoted, the other*

man was "just plain wrong". The group leader, John, could tell that this topic was of immense importance for these two members as their nonverbal language seemed to signal "fight". He tried to defuse the situation and lower the intensity by intervening and using his conflict resolution skills that usually worked. However, while the men participated in the resolution process, neither budged from his initial position, and the group atmosphere remained very tense.

When John asked other group members about their experiences around the conflict, all reported that they had high levels of discomfort, a couple of members just wanted to agree to disagree and move on to something else, and several members reported that they wanted to leave and get away from the conflict. John felt that if he could not reduce the emotional intensity in the room, that there was a real possibility that one or more members might not return to the next session.

John decided to explore members' feelings and reactions around conflict, to provide an opportunity to both members in the conflict to gain insight, and to possibly reduce tension in the group. Members had many fears around conflict because they perceived it as destructive, allowed fears of danger to re-emerge from their childhood experiences, and did not have expectations for positive outcomes from the conflict that was currently in the group. There were even some comments made that suggested a lack of confidence in John's ability to moderate the conflict. Members were fearful that the group would be destroyed. The more members talked, the more intense the atmosphere became on top of the already heightened intensity.

The conflicting group members said that they wanted to group to remain intact, and would just let the conflict go, and not try to resolve it. John knew that it was very unlikely that, if the conflict was suppressed, it would not just go underground but would continue to negatively impact the group.

Students could be asked to brainstorm possible leader actions, and to also list the feelings they think that they would have as the group leader in the vignette. The following discussion/reflection questions can also be fruitful topics: What actions do you use to prevent and/or avoid conflict? To confront? To compromise?

Member–Level Challenges

Presented are the member-level challenges that include difficult or problem member behaviors which are defined as members who display behaviors that are difficult for the leader and group members to manage and are also troubling to the group's process and progress and suggested interventions (Brown, 2006). Next, is the discussion and information about how group leaders may contribute to difficulties for members and for the group. The last topic focuses on group level challenges and interventions. Specific suggestions are provided that can assist the leader to prevent of some behaviors described as difficult, identify some leader behaviors that can be counterproductive; and describe actions to address specific difficult behaviors. Leaders are encouraged to perceive difficult member behaviors as information about the member and/or the group.

Definitions and Descriptions

The difficult group or difficult member is defined here in terms of the group leader's experiencing of the situation or person as disruptive, unhelpful, and in some cases can even be destructive. Rutan and Stone (2001) define difficult groups as those where the leader has "trouble making and sustaining emotional contact", and experience the group as stuck, confusing, boring, frustrating or even unresponsive. Gans and Alonso (1998) use the concept of inter-subjectivity, that is the mutual experiencing of each other's world at the same time, to explain how the group leader and/or other members contribute to the construction of the difficult member, the need that role or difficulty fulfills, and the value of this to the group. They propose that the difficult member can best be understood in terms of the need they fulfill, and that the difficult member is partly a "construction of the whole system" (p. 312). Rutan and Stone (2001) propose that members identified as difficult, such as the mono-polizer and help rejecting complainer, do not exist as such from the self-psychological perspective. This perspective redefines the behavior as the functions that it serves for the person, and for the group. For example, Rutan and Stone write, "The so-called help-rejecting complainer probably does not exist!" (p. 302). They redefine the behavior for this person as a fundamental failure to communicate what help they are looking for, and as empathic failures for both the leader and members.

Goals for troubling behaviors will generally fall into one or more of the following categories: attention, power, control, revenge, protection of the self, yearning for connection or intimacy, fearing connection or intimacy, avoid-ance of emotions and/or emotional intensity., Leaders; by virtue of their training, experience, and personal development; can uncover the possible goal the troubling behavior fulfills, make an empathic connection, be emotionally present so that an empathic response could provide reassurance of caring and safety. This can reassure the member and the group that they will be deeply understood, the possibility of becoming scapegoated can be reduced, and other group members will learn that the group is a safe place, and that the leader is prepared to handle conflict, aggression, and other disquieting behavior.

The *attention* goal is relatively easy to identify as the person will do or say something that brings the group's attention to them such as provocative com-ments, challenging statements, inappropriate jokes, or even prolonged silence and the like. The *power and control goals* may be less easy to identify as the behaviors often have to occur over time to be discerned. The member actions lead to their having influence and power over what the group addresses, who gets to have their issues considered, and indirect challenges to the leader. The *revenge* goal is discerned in that member's behaviors that are demeaning, dismissive, hurtful, or shameful to others. They are seeking revenge for the real or imagined injuries they suffered in their lives, not necessarily in the particular group.

Some member behaviors have the goal of *protection of the self* to prevent being hurt, destroyed or becoming overwhelmed by another person. The goals for some behaviors are either as a *yearning for connections* or intimacy or *fearing connections* and intimacy and so they act to achieve that goal. The final goal presented here is the one that signals that the member's goal is *avoidance of emotions* and/or emotional intensity as a way to ensure that they do not have to experience something that is uncomfortable and may even be considered as dangerous by them.

The Leader's Contributions to Difficulties

Gans and Alonso (1998) feel that the leader can contribute to fostering the construction of the difficult group member in several ways: faulty selection of group members where unsuitability for the group is not identified; incompetent or inappropriate management of group norms, scapegoating and boundary violations; an inability to admit to mistakes; defensiveness when challenged or a refusal to let the members express negative feelings about the leader; and failure to recognize personal limitations. Many of these can be the result of underdeveloped narcissism (Horwitz, 2000), or unresolved narcissistic needs (Gans & Alonso, 1998).

When a group leader becomes defensive that indicates that they are unable to tolerate negative criticisms or of anything that seems to indicate that the leader is not adequate. devaluation. Other leader contributions include being overly nurturing and working to make members like them or feel comfortable, ignoring member's behaviors that are counterproductive to the group's progress, allowing a member to be scapegoated, seeking flattery and compliments from group members, consciously or unconsciously responding favorable to members who affirm the leader's self-perceptions of adequacy and effectiveness, and having an expectation that members will treat them as expert. There are also other more negative behaviors that are contributors such as when the leader uses emotionally abusive behaviors and comments, refusal to admit mistakes and the like, boasts about their personal lives, showing hurt or anger when a member disagrees with them or is dismissive of an intervention, and most negative of all is when the leader does not have the ability to be empathic. Therefore, it is important that the group leader examine their behaviors and attitudes to determine if they have acted to contributed to the difficult member behavior.

Examples of Difficult Member Behavior

Presented are examples of difficult member behaviors and some possible goals to modify the behavior, and some effective leader interventions.

- *Advice giving*. Members are likely to engage in considerable *advice-giving* to try and be helpful. The goal for this behavior is to try to "fix" the issue, problem, or concern.

−Tip: One possible leader intervention is to say to the advice giver: "You really want to be helpful and this is what you can recommend. Another possible leader intervention is to interrupt the advice giving and tell group members that it could be more helpful to report on the feelings the issue or problem or concern aroused.

- *Expert.* The *expert* member may have experience, knowledge, and expertise, but is more likely to just be a know–it–all who is not shy about sharing their thoughts, ideas, solutions, and so on. They too may want to be helpful but are most likely wanting to show off their superiority. A leader intervention could be to respond to the expert and acknowledge that they are trying to be helpful but, as with advice giving, it would be more helpful to the other person to express their thoughts and feelings about that issue instead of trying to "fix" it.

−Tip: A possible leader intervention is to say: "You want to show how to solve the problem (or not make a mistake) based on your knowledge and expertise."

- *Monopolizing.* The *monopolizing* member is often unaware of the impact of their behavior on other members. Their goal is to reduce their anxiety and relieve the tension that can emerge during silence in the group.

−Tip: A possible intervention is to say to the person: "You are taking care of the group and trying to do something that you think would reduce anxiety." Another possible intervention could be to acknowledge that silence can be uncomfortable and to open that discussion up to the group as to their responses to prolonged silence.

- *Storytelling.* The *storytelling* behavior is often appreciated in the beginning stage of the group because other members can focus on this member instead of on their personal concerns as the story gives an illusion that the group is working. The storyteller is also anxious, and is engaging in some social convention behavior by providing extensive details.

−Tip: An intervention can be to interrupt the story and tell the member that while they want to ensure that they are fully understood, it is much more important to know and understand their feelings about the matter than to hear the details.

- *Sullen.* The *sullen* member is often an involuntary member, such as a court order participant. The sullen member is present in body, and brings negativity, hostility, and suppressed anger to the group. They may not be openly defiant but is not pleased or open to being in the group. There can be resentment for their circumstances, a grudge for life's experiences or for a particular person's unfairness that can be displaced on the leader and other group members, and a lack of commitment or participation in the group. The goal for this behavior is usually revenge for what they have experienced.

—Tip: A possible leader intervention can be to ask other group members to report on their feelings about unfair treatment, being forced to do something they do not want to do, feeling trapped, and so on. Generate a discussion about the universality of these experiences and the resulting feelings. Be sure to have each member speak for what they feel, and to block advice giving.

- *Withdrawal.* Although the sullen member may exhibit withdrawal behaviors, there are other reasons for the behavior such as being a signal a need to protect oneself from something that is dangerous or threatening, either in the group or emerging from within the person that is triggered by group events, or by group members as part of transference. The primary goal for this behavior is defense of the self.

—Tip: A possible intervention is to directly ask the member for input, or if there is something happening in the group that is producing their reaction.

- *Yes ... but.* This behavior generally results from frustration at self or at others as they are seeking answers or solutions, has a particular desired outcome in mind, cannot generate actions or alternatives that would seem to be feasible, or that would guarantee the desired outcome, and is closed to the possibilities suggested by others. The goal is to get the desired answer, which is elusive.

—Tip: An intervention would be to simply empathically respond that it is frustrating to not get answers that seem to fit.

- *Sarcasm.* Sarcastic remarks are indirect ways to express thoughts and feelings, and these can be very hurtful to the receiver who has few effective responses available. The speaker is fearful of the results, such as an attack, if they should voice their real feelings or thoughts, and hides them. The goal is to not have to accept responsibility for what can be hurtful to someone else.

—Tip: An intervention would be to ask the speaker to report on their thoughts and feelings even if they were to say that they were just joking.

Leaders are encouraged to quickly intervene when any of these behaviors occur as these can be very hurtful to group members. Other strategies include prevention actions.

Constructive Prevention Strategies

Preparing members to maximize the group experience for personal benefit will do much to reduce the difficult and counterproductive behaviors. Preparation includes informing members of expected behavior, and guidelines for relating and participation. Other preparation would describe behaviors such as expressing important thoughts and feelings as they emerge in sessions, and taking personal responsibility for their progress and input such as making "I" statements instead of general and vague ones.

Counterproductive Leader Interventions

There are also some interventions to avoid as they are likely to be counterproductive. These apply in both the group as a whole, and individual member situations. Examples include dismissing the behavior as trivial or unimportant, expressing anger or annoyance, intended humorous sarcasm as this can be easily misunderstood by group members, lecturing, labeling the group or member, and saying things that seem blaming or critical and can be shaming. Other leader behaviors that affect the group are misuse of the leader's role with the intent to intimidate, for the leader to become defensive, or for the leader to fail to monitor their countertransference to ensure that unresolved personal issues are not influencing the choice of action (Cohen, 2000; Gans & Alonso, 1998; Horwitz, 2000; Livingston & Livingston, 1998; Schermer, 2000; Wright, 2000).

A Deviant Group Member

A deviant group member can have a significant negative impact on the group and its process and progress, on individual group members, and can present a challenge to the group leader. Yalom and Leszcz (2005) proposed that the deviant group member runs the risk of being harmed for example, becomes the group scapegoat. *Deviant* for this discussion refers to a group member who is deviant "because of their interpersonal behavior in the group sessions, not because of a deviant lifestyle or history" (p. 244); one whose "behavior or characteristics are unambiguously undesirable" (Hutchison, Abrams, & DeMoura, 2013, p. 344); one who is disliked (Marques & Paez, 1994); or one who has a demeanor that makes them unsuitable for the group (Burlingame, Cox, Davis, Layne, & Gleave, 2011; Jetten & Hornsey, 2014). These group members present threats to the group process (McNair & Corazzini, 1994), disagree with group norms so that the group experiences greater dissonance (Matz & Wood, 2005), are less likable (Hichy, Marit, & Capozza, 2008; Morrison & Miller, 2008), and lead to decreased group cohesion (Burlingame et al., 2011). The deviant group member is an outlier for the group's identity (Hutchison et al., 2013) and shared norms or values (Matz & Wood, 2005) and can exhibit self-absorbed behaviors and attitudes (Kearns & Brown, 2016).

Importance and Rational for Identification

Groups are more likely to achieve cohesion when there is trust among group members; when each member has a shared commitment to the group and its goals as well as to himself or herself; when there is a willingness to give and receive feedback; when there is a sense of safety, where the real self can be disclosed and seen with the confidence that it will be accepted; and where there is a harmonious holding and containing environment. This stage of group development provides the climate where considerable growth, development, and healing can occur. Agazarian (1997) postulated that groups become cohesive around shared similarities and fail to be-come cohesive because of perceived differences that are important for the particular group members. Thus an important variable when organizing and composing a group can be the similarities among potential group members. *Similarity* is defined here as the extent to which the members of a group are seen as similar in terms of relevant group attributes (Hutchison et al., 2013; Hutchison, Jetten, & Gutierrez, 2011), which deepens the meaning and intent of similarity, because the perceived similarities for a particular group move beyond commonalities of visible characteristics, such as race/ethnicity, age, or gender; the commonalities around a condition or issue that is the purpose for the group, such as substance abuse or divorce; or the commonalities for coworkers or peers. These superficial and often visible characteristics may be helpful, in some ways, to allow members to connect in the beginning of the group but do not address the need members have to connect around deeper meaningful and significant similarities. The concept of the deviant group member and his or her early identification is important because of his or her negative effect on the group and its members, such as the tendency for the group to derogate the member perceived as deviant (Hutchison et al., 2013), for the member to be psychologically isolated (Hutchison et al., 2013; Jetten et al., 2011), for the member to be scapegoated (Yalom & Leszcz, 2005), and for the group members to spend time trying to isolate and protect the group from the deviant group member. Groups that do not or cannot use screening to ferret out the deviancy prior to composing the group can be especially vulnerable to having to manage and contain the disruptions to the group process and progress. It is also possible that the screening process, when implemented, will not identify the potential deviant. The use of an instrument such as the Group Selection Questionnaire's Demeanor Scale (Burlingame et al., 2011) would be helpful in identifying the deviant prior to his or her being placed in a group. This discussion focuses on identification of group members' behaviors, attitudes, and feelings that can suggest deviancy, the various responses groups as a whole can exhibit to the person considered as deviant, some potential impacts on individual group members, and leader strategies.

Deviant Behavior and Demeanor

Deviant in this discussion means that the person is behaving in such a way that is displeasing to the other group members; is out of synch; or is different in a way that could produce rejection, exclusion, or psychological isolation and where the group expends considerable time and effort trying to make the deviant conform to the core values of the group and exhibit acceptable behavior, opinions, attitudes, and the like. Deviant behavior has been described as avoiding verbal arguments, holding back from speaking in groups, avoiding sharing feelings, and not seeing the group as potentially helpful. The items on Burlingame's Demeanor Scale include feeling left out and/or ignored, suppressing negative emotions, making inappropriate disclosures, arguing for argument's sake, talking over others, and showing domineering behaviors. Some typical behaviors that can be indicative of a possible deviant group member are seen in the following descriptions.

- The know-it-all group member, who has an answer or solution for everything talked about in the group.
- The member who exhibits a tendency to assume a "devil's advocate" role by not providing perceptions, feelings, responses, and the like, but almost always saying something like, "I'd like to play the devil's advocate in this discussion – not that this is my perception, but just saying".
- A member who is always or almost always is ready to give advice as to what a group member or the leader should or ought to do.
- The member who presents their life experiences as justification for knowing what needs to be done, usually by others.
- Boasting about accomplishments, material objects, or anything that makes them feel important and superior to other group members.
- Members who lacking insight and seems unwilling to explore their selves.
- Members who demonstrate little or no empathy toward others but expect it from others.
- A member or members who tend to exhibit indifference to others' concerns and their impact on others.
- The member who talks over others, finish other members' thoughts, and interrupt to take the conversation in a different direction.
- Members seeking admiration and responding favorably to flattery.
- Members who make denigrating and/or disparaging comments to and about others.

The deviant group member can have a negative impact on the group and its members with their behaviors that may also be indicative of considerable self-absorption. However, it may not be possible for the group leader to remove that member or to suggest another placement that could be more effective for them. In cases like this where the deviant group member has to remain in the group, the group leader has the task of protecting other group members from the deviant member's destructive behaviors and attitudes. One suggestion for managing this extremely difficult situation is for the group leader to have the group focus on more cognitive topics rather than feelings. Leaders can also block some negative behaviors, and reframe the comments, or redirect the session.

Summary

This chapter focused on describing some behaviors and attitudes of group members that can present difficulties for the group leader and for the group. While these difficulties cannot always be prevented, the group leader can help the group manage these with their understanding of how the behavior and/or attitudes impact and affect the group and its members as well as the particular group member. Suggestions for managing some difficulties were provided.

References

Agazarian, Y. (1997). *Systems-Centered Therapy for Groups*. New York: Guilford Press.

Brown, N. W. (2006). *Coping with Infuriating, Mean, Critical People*. Westpoint, CT: Praeger.

Burlingame, G., Cox, J., Davis, R., Layne, C., & Gleave, R. (2011). The group selection questionnaire: Further refinements in group member selection. *Group Dynamics: Theory, Research, and Practice*, 15(1), 60–74.

Cohen, B. D. (2000) Intersubjectivity and narcissism in group psychotherapy: How feedback works. *International Journal of Group Psychotherapy*, 50(2), 163–179.

Gans, J. S., & Alonso, A. (1998). Difficult patients: Their construction in group therapy. *International Journal of Group Psychotherapy*, 48, 311–326.

Hichy, Z., Marit, S., & Capozza, D. (2008). Pro-norm and anti-norm deviants: A test of the subjective group dynamics model. *European Journal of Social Psychology*, 48(1), 641–644.

Horwitz, L. (2000) Narcissistic leadership in psychotherapy groups, *International Journal of Group Psychotherapy*, 50(2), 219–235.

Hutchison, P., Abrams, D., & DeMoura, G. (2013). Corralling the ingroup: Deviant derogation and perception of group variability. *Journal of Social Psychology*, 153, 334–350.

Hutchison, P., Jetten, J., & Gutierrez, R. (2011). Deviant but desirable: Perceived group variability and reactions to atypical group members. *Journal of Experimental Social Psychology*, 47, 1155–1161.

Jetten, J., & Hornsey, M. (2014). Deviance and dissent in groups. *Annual Review of Psychology*, 65, 461–485.

Jetten, J., Iyer, A., Hutchison, P., & Hornsey, M. (2011). Debating deviance: Responding to those who fall from grace. In J. Jetten & M. Hornsey (Eds.), *Rebels in Groups* (pp. 117–134). Oxford: Wiley-Blackwell.

Kearns, K., & Brown, N. (2016). Comparisons between newcomers, chronic relapsers & endurers attending an AA program. *Journal of Groups in Addictions and Recovery*, 11, 156–165.

Kernberg, O. F. (1990). *Borderline Conditions and Pathological Narcissism*. Northvale, NJ: Aronson.

Kohut, H. (1977) *The Restoration of the Self*. Madison, CT: International Universities.

Kohut, H., & Wolf, E. S. (1978). The disorders of the self and their treatment: An outline. *The International Journal of Psychoanalysis*, 59(4), 413–425.

Livingston, M., & Livingston, L. L. (1998). Conflict and aggression in group psychotherapy: A self psychological vantage point. *International Journal of Group Psychotherapy*, 48, 381–391.

Marques, J., & Paez, D. (1994). The "black sheep effect": Social categorization, rejection of ingroup deviancy, and perception of group variability. *European Review of Social Psychology*, 5, 37–58.

Matz, D., & Wood, W. (2005). Cognitive dissonance in groups: The consequences of disagreement. *Journal of Personality and Social Psychology*, 88(1), 22–37.

McNair, R., & Corazzini, J. (1994). Client factors influencing group therapy dropout. *Psychotherapy: Theory, Research, Practice, Training*, 31, 352–362.

Morrison, K., & Miller, D. (2008). Distinguishing between silent and vocal minorities: Not all deviants feel marginal. *Journal of Personality and Social Psychology*, 94, 871–872.

Reich, W. (1972). *Character Analysis*. New York: Simon and Schuster.

Rutan, S. J. & Stone, N. W. (2001). *Psychodynamic Groups Psychotherapy* (3rd edition). New York: Guilford Press.

Schermer, V. (2000) Contributions of object relations theory and self psychology to relational psychology and group psychotherapy. *International Journal of Group Psychotherapy*, 50(2), 199–217.

Stone, W. N. (1992). The place of self psychology in group psychotherapy: A status Report. *International Journal of Group Psychotherapy*, 42, 335–350.

Wright, F. (2000) The use of the self in group leadership: A relational perspective. *International Journal of Group Psychotherapy*. 50(2), 181–198.

Yalom, I., & Leszcz, M. (2005). *The Theory and Practice of Group Psychotherapy*. New York: Basic Books.

10 Intangible and Unseen Forces that Impact the Group

There are some intangible and unseen forces that impact the group's functioning, but little is available in the literature to guide beginning group leaders in identification of these, or constructive interventions. It is reasonable to accept that group members (transference) and the leader (countertransference) bring their previous life experiences to the group in some way; that these experiences have influences on behavior, attitudes, feelings, and relationships; that there may not always be conscious awareness of these and how they influence personal perceptions and responses (resistance); and that their intangible and unseen nature impact the group. However these intangible forces are termed, they should not be overlooked, discounted, or ignored. This discussion uses the terms resistance, transference, and countertransference.

Group Resistance

While resistance is always expected in a group, there are times when the leader has to determine if the resistance is for individual(s) or for the group as a whole. The following vignette presents a scenario that shows how complex that decision could be.

Vignette

> The group had started off with much promise and Duncan, the group leader, was pleased with the progress so far. He felt that members were gaining benefits from the group that would encourage them to stick to their plans to combat their abuse of alcohol. He wasn't naive with unrealistic expectations, as he had worked with many clients having this condition over the years and knew that their challenges would not be easily overcome, and there was much hard work to be done. But he was encouraged because of the behaviors in the group, and their reported behaviors outside the group that seemed to be verified by family members.
>
> During the sixth session, Duncan noticed that several topics introduced by members did not seem finished. As soon as one member finished talking, a perfunctory response was provided by another member, but then that member, or another one,

DOI: 10.4324/9781003329787-10

went on to talk about something else. Duncan made a mental note to himself to pay attention to this and bring it to the group's attention if it happened again. The next session was a repeat of the previous one, and Duncan did intervene with a group process comment. The members reflected on what they were doing, and possible reasons, but it was not long before they were back into the skittering pattern. The same happened the next session where Duncan tried another group process comment. Members tried to be reflective about what they were doing but continued the established pattern. There was no new material in what the members were talking about, and they really seemed to try to cooperate with Duncan's interventions.

Resistance is not irrational, a weakness, or wrong, it has an important function and purpose, as described by some theorists. Sigmund Freud (1936 [1926]) described resistance as that used by the client to protect against the pain of recognizing unbearable ideas. Anna Freud's book *The Ego and the Mechanisms of Defense* (Freud, 1946) expanded the concept of defenses used as resistance to include their use in everyday life. Reich (1972) felt that individuals use their character traits, or characterological armor, as resistance, and Hartman (1958) thought of it as protection for the ego. However, all of these definitions relate to individuals, but these can combine to become group level resistance. That is, individual members may be resisting and resisting for different reasons, but the collective result is group level resistance. In psychoanalytic terms, resistance is the client's attempt to block or repress anxiety-provoking memories and insights from entering conscious awareness.

Activity

Think of an event or situation or person where you were resistant. Image your resistance and describe it. After sharing the image, identify three or more elements involved that aroused your resistance such as sensitivity about the topic or person, feeling attached or overwhelmed, feeling inadequate or shame or embarrassment or chagrin. Either write about your experience or share in small groups.

Identification

A group resistance can emerge at any time during the life of the group and can be unexpected and disconcerting. The leader may not recognize the group resistance at first because each member is expressing the resistance in different ways, and there can be a tendency to focus on individual resistance. Clues to possible group as a whole resistance can be the following.

- The leader is puzzled or confused about what is taking place in the session.
- Interventions and suggestions are ignored, discounted, or are ineffective.
- Several members get confused or misunderstand what the leader says or means.

- Group members become snappish and cranky with each other, and this is a change from their usual behavior.
- The discussion in the session is unfocused and wide ranging, usually on outside the group topics.
- The session feels unsettling to the leader, and/or to group members.
- Formerly participating members are quiet, reserved or may appear to be withdrawn.

The group leader can consider if the group as a whole is resisting something about the group including the leader. Following are some suggested signals that there is group level resistance rather than individual resistance.

- After the group has met for several sessions, the current session could be described as "milling around". No one topic seems to be of interest, there are numerous topics introduced that could lead to constructive work, but no one picks up on them.
- The group starts and continues social chit-chat. No one seems to be upset that no work is being done.
- A member is scapegoated.
- Every attempt the leader makes to bring the discussion to the here and now is rebuffed and members continue to focus on there and then topics.
- All suggestions from the leader are met with a "yes ... but" response.
- Whatever the leader says is complimented and/or agreed with by the members.
- Members are obviously ignoring the leader.
- The group seems out of sorts. Members are cranky and grumpy.
- Group members make discounting and devaluing comments about the leader.
- The group reports feeling "stuck".
- The leader cannot intervene successfully to move the group to another topic, they keep returning to the same topic even though members seem, or say, they are tired of rehashing the same material.

The challenge then becomes to identify what the group is resisting about the group. The first step can be to identify if the defenses being used would be fight or flight.

Thorenson (1972) proposed three categories for group resistance: flight defenses, fight defenses and group manipulation defenses. Flight defenses are employed to avoid dealing with intense feeling aroused in the group, fight defenses are employed to deflect attention, generally in an attacking way and group manipulation defenses are used to protect oneself against deep involvement. Some examples may be helpful. *Flight defenses* can be inferred when the group continues to resist being present-centered. Most, or all, group members participate in the flight although each may use a different defense. Some member defenses that may indicate group flight defenses are intellectualization, generalizing, projecting, rationalization, and withdrawal. *Fight* defenses are often employed to resist challenging the leader, to avoid bringing the attention to them and so they challenge each other. Some behaviors that can signal fight defense are competition with the leader, open skepticism of process and progress of the group, attacking each other and/or intense questioning of each other. *Group manipulation* defenses can be used to protect members against intimacy. The threat is that by becoming close they fear that they will not be found to be adequate and will be rejected. Behaviors that characterize group manipulation are: forming alliances, rescuing, band-aiding, and having an "identified patient" to fix. Members are individually and collectively resisting intimacy, being manipulated or controlled, having the "self" be known, rejection, allowing conflict to emerge, becoming enmeshed, being abandoned, or being destroyed.

Tuning in to Group Resistance

Leaders may find that the first sign of group resistance is by experiencing a generalized disquiet, or sense that they are missing something taking place in the group. The leader simply feels that something is awry. Leader strategies for recognizing group level resistance include identifying the session's theme, noting stress points, where resistance seems to be especially strong, attending to shifts in participation, direction, and the like, recognizing behaviors related to group stages, free association, and metaphor analysis.

The session's theme can be a signal. The theme is the underlying thread that ties the discussed topics together such as most of the topics discussed were outside of the group issues and concerns. *Shifts in level and extent of participation* can be signals that the group members are uncomfortable with something in the group and so they meet the discomfort with increased or decreased participation or bring the level of participation up to be somewhat trivial. *Continual discussions of there and then topics* although some may be significant for the group member can suggest that it is less dangerous to talk about things other than what is happening in the group between members and with the group leader.

Possible Reasons for Resistance

There are many possible reasons for the group as a whole resistance; members feel or sense that there is danger, empathic failures have occurred, there may be suppressed conflict, it could be reflective of the stage of group development, and there may be individual reasons.

Bion (1961) and others who developed group as a whole understanding, termed these group actions as fight or flight. The group is protecting itself from *real or imagined danger* and these are the strategies they use. There is no conscious collusion among members to resist, no discussion about the real or imagined danger, or an understanding of what they collectively are doing.

The group leader's task is to determine what the real or imagined danger may be, and to do it for the entire group and not focus on individual resistance except to link these in order to understand the group's resistance. The leader needs to reflect on previous group sessions, the stage of group development, and incorporate individual members' needs and issues into their deliberations. This is also where some attention to group process could be of assistance.

Reflecting on the present and previous sessions allows the leader to recall if there was an event, *missed empathic failures,* or an overlooked opportunity that could be contributing to the group's feeling of danger. For example, is conflict being suppressed, minimized, or ignored? How the group manages conflict could lead to feelings of danger as conflict is not being worked through. The uncertainty about when and how it could or will emerge can lead to feeling unsafe. Another example could be that empathic failures occurred for several members over several sessions, and these were not repaired. Members can then wonder when they and others will be failed again and be very fearful of the impact on them.

The *stage of group development* can also be a factor in group resistance. For example, since conflict is a characteristic of stage 2, the group may be fearful of having conflict in the group, or of challenging the leader. Several, or all group members could be fearful of intimacy and help produce group resistance for stages 1 and 3. The group could be resisting termination if the group is in the ending stage. It could be helpful for leaders to remember characteristic behaviors for each group stage to see if this is a part of the explanation for the resistance.

Individual members' needs and issues may also be factors in the group resistance, especially when there are deep similarities among members. The leader can link these as part of understanding the resistance. For example, although their experiences were different, several group members could have issues around betrayal, rejection, and the resulting pain. Thus, when the group seems on the verge of becoming more intimate, connected, and involved, their fears about these previous experiences emerge, and collectively members ward off the potential danger by resistance.

Addressing Group Resistance

Once the leader identifies the presence of group resistance the next task is to decide what, if anything, to do to address that. Leaders will find it helpful to avoid attacking the resistance or the group, becoming defensive, or do anything that suggests that the leader is disappointed or is blaming the group. There are some behaviors that will, in the long run, be constructive. The leader will find it most helpful to leave the resistance alone especially in groups like short term groups. But it is also helpful to stay in contact with the resistance and at some point bring the resistance to the group's attention by a carefully timed group process comment. By not doing anything that suggests that the group is wrong, or to try to minimize or eliminate the resistance, the group leader reassures members that they are in charge of what they want to disclose and that they are empowered to be in charge of their safety. *Staying in contact* with the resistance provides leaders with information about the individual members' issues about their safety. *A process comment* can make visible the resistance without suggestions that resistance is wrong. *Making process commentary* highlights the resistance without demanding that they stop resisting.

It is not uncommon for groups to resist letting the real self be seen for fear of rejection conflict emerging, their becoming connected or intimate, or of challenging the group leader. The fear that the leader and other group members will see *the "real self" and reject* it can lead some members to exhibit considerable resistance. They are convinced on some level that if others see their real self, that will be seen as inadequate and thus will be destroyed. It is not unusual for group members to *resist conflict emergence* in the group as their past experiences have led them to believe that conflict is unpleasant, destructive, and harmful. The fear of *intimacy* can produce strong resistance which is usually tied to previous experiences where they experienced rejection, or betrayal, or abandonment, or destruction, or enmeshment and the like.

These situations describe an environment where individual resistance is not an adequate explanation for what is happening.

Use of Group Process Commentary

Incorporating group process at this point would mean attending to the here and now interactions among group members, to what the group as a whole was doing or not doing when the resistance occurred or was noticed, the theme and feeling tone of the group as a whole for that session, and the internal experiencing of the group leader. Putting all of this information together can usually help identify what is, or what may be, resisted by all members in some form.

Some general threats to members' safety that can produce group resistance include the following.

- Resisting intimacy – members' past experiences and insecurities about tolerating closeness and connection can produce this resistance.
- Resisting becoming known to others for fear of rejection.
- Resisting disclosing shameful secrets or unacceptable parts of self.
- Resisting for fear of being hurt, abandoned or destroyed.
- Resisting challenging the leader.
- Resisting conflict emerging among members.

Identifying the possible threat can provide the leader with some ideas for intervention strategies. Unlike what is recommended for resistance by individuals which is that the resistance be noted and left alone, group resistance calls for some intervention by the leader. Leaving group resistance unaddressed can cause the group to feel even less safe for members, prevent the group from engaging in productive work, and retard group progress.

After identification of a possible threat, the leader should take into consideration the stage of group development, and the emotional state of members, such as their emotional fragility or emotional maturity. A good intervention is a group process comment about what the group is doing or not doing, but not trying to interpret the behavior or to name it as resistance. Possible reasons or hypotheses can be suggested, but the group should not be presented with an interpretation. The comment and possible reasons can be explored in the group.

However, making group process comment in the beginning stage of group is usually not advisable as members are still getting use to each other and the leader, the social convention taboo about speaking openly about observed behavior is still in effect, and group members can feel very threatened or criticized by these comments. Groups in stages 2 and on can be more receptive and ready to make constructive use of group process commentary.

These situations describe an environment where individual resistance is not an adequate explanation for what is happening.

Activity: Practice Group Process Commentary

Directions:

1 Divide the class into small groups of 3–5 students and tell them that this is a practice group commentary activity. Tell them the directions below and ask if there are any questions.
2 Distribute the activity.
3 Ask students to first identify the group resistance and second, to write their group process comment individually.
4 Ask students to discuss their answers in their small groups.
5 Have each group report out on what was identified as the resistance noting any differences between members.
6 Ask for examples of group process comments from group members.

(Note: A suggested resistance is given below each situation.).
Group situations:

1 The group composed of 8 young adults aged 22–35 is meeting for the eighth session. Group members all seem to be from the same culture/

ethnic/racial group and are either employed or in college. This group session begins with the leader asking if there is unfinished business from the previous session or if members are bringing something important and/or urgent to the group that day. No one has anything to say.

- *(Resistance – intimacy)*

2   Near the beginning of the third session, members ask the leader personal questions about their family and background.

- *(Resistance – trust and safety)*

3   About halfway through the third session a member suggests that the group appoint a chair to conduct the future sessions, and that they select topics to discuss in advance of the sessions. Other members openly agree with the suggestion or nod their heads.

- *(Resistance – challenge to the leader)*

4   The group spends much of the fifth session talking about politics. No one appears displeased with the discussion, and it looks like it may continue for the remainder of the session.

- *(Resistance – politics in the group- unfair/unequal treatment)*

Scapegoating

Agazarian (1997) notes that "the group creates a scapegoat role to contain the differences that the group system is not yet ready to integrate" (p. 191). The scapegoat serves a purpose for the group, and is a role that is uncomfortable and nonconscious for that person except when the leader consciously accepts the role. This person, or the leader, becomes the repository and/or target for members' personal and unacceptable thoughts, fantasies, needs, projections, transference, and displacement. The person is the "identified patient" in need of fixing so that members do not have to work on their personal issues, concerns and the like; or the person who speaks of the negative or unacceptable perceptions or perspectives that members cannot or are unwilling to openly verbalize. The scapegoat usually assumes the role unintentionally when they speak the unacceptable, exhibit behavior that arouses indignation or irritation, is active or in the spotlight, is out of sync with most other members, and so on.

Following are some indices that scapegoating may be present in the group.

- The group continually focuses on one member and tries to "fix" that member's concerns.
- Group members become irritated, upset, and/or critical of one member or the leader; and can express negative feelings toward the person.

- The group leader is continually challenged in the meeting, or over several sessions, about a member's behavior.
- A member is labeled by several members such as being uncaring, detached, different from other members, and so on.

The leader must intervene to protect the scapegoated member, and to keep the group from being divided. Cohesion cannot be built unless all group members are accepted and valued. The focus here is on the scapegoated member and how to better protect the person and to promote more group cohesion. Let's examine four possible examples of scapegoating.

- *Center of attention.* This person will usually have a significant problem or crisis that keeps them in the group's spotlight and members can become irritated feeling that the member gets all of the attention.

  —Tip: After the first one or two incidences, the leader should block the story and also acknowledge the validity of the member's concern or problem, and how members want to be helpful; but also point out that it may be more helpful if group members would respond empathically instead of giving advice, and/or ask questions.

- *Cranky and attacking.* When group members become cranky, critical, and/or attacking, the group is probably acting on suppressed conflict, either among members or with the leader. However, if a group member becomes the target for the suppressed conflict and receives much or most of the negative comments, then that person is the scapegoat.

  —Tip: Leaders must act quickly to block the attacking or criticizing behavior, and to protect the targeted member. One of the following two questions can be posed to the group. Are the feelings expressed (by the scapegoated member) shared or are similar to feelings other members have but have not expressed? Could it be that this member is challenged so that members don't have to challenge the leader?

- *Challenge to the leader.* Leaders can be scapegoated and serve as containers for the negative feelings members have about themselves. The leader may even be termed as intimidating, uncaring, distant, or unhelpful. What members may be trying to convey is their desire to become less dependent on the leader, some self-criticism, or what they wish the leader to be or do.

  —Tip: The leader should listen carefully to the challenges and determine what are the disguised needs, wishes and desires that are contained in the challenge. The level of the leader's personal development can assist in understanding if they are serving as the group's container of these unspoken wishes and the like.

Of course, the leader needs to examine their behavior to assess the validity of the challenges, and make changes where needed. If the challenge is not valid, the leader must respond carefully and with empathy, but should not become defensive.

- *Labeling comments.* These behaviors can be the most overt signals for scapegoating. Labels are usually pejorative or judgmental, even when stated in a manner or with a stated intent of being helpful. The hidden or unconscious intent is to place the blame, unacceptable personal feelings, and so on, outside of oneself and to redefine the problem as the scapegoat's need to be fixed. It's much easier to work on someone else than it is to work on oneself.

—Tip: The leader can set a norm and culture of asking group members to report on their thoughts, feelings, reactions, and so on, when responding to other members. If this has been established, then when labeling occurs, the leader can intervene with a statement or request that it would be more helpful to tell the labeled member the impact and/or reactions that emerge when experiencing the member's behavior. For example, if a member was labeled as angry, the leader could intervene and ask other group members to report on their feelings and other reactions to the labeled member's behavior instead of labeling them as angry.

Competition

Competition in the group is to be expected but need not be destructive or a problem. Group members compete for attention; for admiration; being the most needy; to be considered as unique and special; for power, dominance, control; and for getting their needs met. The most common and obvious competition is for the leader's liking, approval, and as being favored, much like what happens in a family where siblings compete for parental favor. On occasion, there will be members who compete with the leader for control of the group, which is more difficult to identify and manage. The leader's countertransference, unresolved issues and unfinished business, and undeveloped narcissism all play critical roles in how competition is managed. Some member behaviors that suggest competition is likely present in the group include frequent boasts and brags, playing one-upmanship, using put downs, constantly agreeing with the leader, developing greater needs and dependency, asking the leader for favors, and/or special sessions outside the group, protecting the leader from attacks and/or criticism, or trying to become the leader's assistant.

It is important that leaders stay aware of their possible countertransference issues so that they do not become a part of competitive behavior in the group, or unwittingly cause problems by seeming to have favorite group members.

Seduction

Seduction is a form of manipulation used to gain control of others, or to get what the person wants and desires, and/or to show that person's superiority. There can be seductive behaviors in the group such as flirting, being provocative, pushing to get someone to disclose more than they want to disclose, rush to rescue or protect someone, pretend to care, or try to have a unique, special, personal, and exclusive relationship with members and/or the leader.

It is a misuse of the power differential when leaders seduce members, and if the seduction becomes erotic or sexual, there is also an ethical violation. All ethical codes prohibit a sexual relationship, and some recognize the dangers of a romantic relationship, and for a coercive one. What about the reverse situation where a member tries to seduce the leader? Leaders should learn to recognize seductive behavior and have sufficient personal development to be able to resist it.

It is considerably more difficult to prevent seduction among group members because they are less likely to have the knowledge, awareness, and level of personal development that the leader has that would prevent their responding to it. That is why it is the leader's responsibility to stay aware of what may be happening and to try and intervene before it becomes troublesome.

Very Difficult Group Members

There are members who have serious developmental issues that can challenge the leader, disrupt the group and its progress, be difficult to identify as such even with screening, and there are few or no interventions that will work. Group members who have any of the following fall into this category: borderline personality disorder (BPD), narcissistic personality disorder (NPD), antisocial/psychopathic disorder, or uncontrolled rage that can explode at any time are some examples of the really difficult group member, primarily because they were undiagnosed before putting them in the group. This can be particularly true of the NPD member who tends to remain unidentified as such for a long time, and it is only through sustained contact over time that the group leader identifies him/her through the leader's persistent feelings and reactions (Kernberg 1990; Brown, 1998). These difficult group members can exert an unconscious corrosiveness on the group where the leader will not make much headway on building safety and trust, and can seem to have to constantly work through conflicts. These members make the group appear to be difficult, and a group only needs to have one such member for there to be a negative impact. The group and the leader can spend a disproportionate amount of time trying to contain a difficult member, and this reduces the time they can spend working on more important issues. The leader is not ineffective but can feel so if these difficult group members go unidentified as such.

The most difficult thing for group leaders to accept under these circumstances is that there is little or nothing that can be done that will be effective for the group. Even if the member were to leave or be removed from the group, the damage has been done and the therapeutic alliance compromised. Screening and diagnosis prior to the group's beginning is the best solution, but this may not be possible for reasons listed in the chapter on planning.

Transference and Countertransference

There are several definitions for transference, and all trying to give substance to an abstract concept that cannot be directly observed, only inferred. Transference involves childhood memories that are stored, mental representations of significant others, affect, relationships with significant others in childhood, unconscious interpretations of childhood relationships and events, and application of these to new encounters. Hoffer (1952) defines transference as any form of object relationship, that is images of people that were experienced as infants and children, Freud's (1953 [1912]) concept of transference emphasized childhood fantasies and conflicts with parents. Andersen and Berk (1998) propose a social-cognitive model for transference derived from empirical studies that transference is not limited to therapy, it also occurs in everyday life. The social-cognitive model of transference does not discount the unconscious nature, but seems to suggest that, because it is so common, a group leader should expect it to be an integral part of all relationships in the group. Extending this perspective to the group allows the leader to observe group members' behaviors and attitudes displayed in the group as being reflective of those outside of the groups.

Transference occurs when group members perceive the group leader and/or other group members as having characteristics like someone they knew in a previous relationship, usually a relationship from the family of origin. This perception leads to their responding and reacting to them as if they were this person. This happens on an unconscious level and the person is not responded to or reacted to in terms of objective reality that is, as they really are, but in terms of the "old" relationship.

Fuertes et al. (2013) categorize transference as positive, negative, or sexualized. Positive transference occurs when enjoyable aspects from the past are projected onto someone or something in the present. Negative transference is the opposite of positive in that the feelings projected in the present are negative or hostile. Sexualized transference are projections of intimacy, attraction, reverence, romantic or sensual. Past relationships that are sources for transference can be associated with the target for the present relationship as one of the following.

- Parental where the target is perceived as powerful, wise, authoritative, and/or protective.

- Maternal where the target is perceived as loving, influential and/or comforting.
- Sibling relationships that produced competition and/or envy.
- Non-familial relationships at any point in one's life that result in idealization or stereotyping.
- Erotic where the target is focus for sexual attraction or otherwise sexualized.

Leader responses to hypothesized or perceived transference to them in short term therapy are most effective when the following are used: empathic responding, refraining from analysis or highlighting, and using links. When a group leader suspects that a member's responses or relating style could be transference, a reflective or empathic response can be helpful. For example, perceived member transference could reflect the member's parental or maternal relationship such as their seeing the leader as authoritative or comforting. It is strongly recommended that the leader refrain from any analyzing, or labeling, or highlighting of the transference as this is likely to be threatening and not well received. Analysis is helpful after a strong therapeutic relationship is developed for that member and for the group which is what happens in long term therapy where analysis will be more helpful. What can be helpful is to use linking to propose associations with previous people and events that have been disclosed in the group, and/or interpersonal relationships with the leader and other group members. This focus is observable by all group members who could then provide consensual validation.

It is also possible that the transference is the member's expression for what they want or need. For example, if the transference is parental, the member may be asking for protection, if maternal they may be asking for comfort and so on with the other types of relationships. It is not unusual for sibling, non-familial, and erotic transference to appear is any group and at any time.

An understanding of transference helps promote a deeper and better understanding of countertransference presented in the next section.

Countertransference

Countertransference is defined as the group leader's reactions and feelings toward a group member that is unconscious and can be detrimental to therapy (Ackerman et al., 2001; Beutler et al., 2002; Leahy, 2003). Fritscher (2021) identified four types of countertransference: subjective, objective, positive and negative. Subjective countertransference occurs because of the group leader's unresolved issues from the family of origin and other past experiences. Fritscher identifies objective countertransference as the therapist reaction to the client's maladaptive behaviors. Brown (2021) uses another definition that perceives objective countertransference as the leader acting as the container for the group's feelings where a realization and understanding of these helps to suggest a response or intervention. Fritscher's definitions for positive and negative countertransference focus on the therapist's actions such as overly identifying with a client or being overly critical or disapproving. It is helpful to think of these descriptions of positive and/or negative countertransference as signals to the group leader that they may be reacting and responding to the group or group members in a harmful way.

Rosenberg et al. (2021) provide the following examples of the group leader's possible countertransference.

- Excessive identification with the disclosures and sharing too many personal stories in the misguided attempt to show that they understand or have had the same experiences.
- Tries to "fix it", provides advice or indirectly tells the members what they should or ought to do.
- Pushes group members to take actions because the leader thinks that these are helpful to members.
- Relates to group members outside of the therapy room in a social or personal way.
- Inappropriately discloses personal information.
- Is overly critical or overly supportive of group members.
- Does not maintain proper and consistent psychological boundaries with group members.

Promoting the Corrective Emotional Experience

The theoretical framework of the group leader will determine how they will choose to work with the information about members' issues around family of origin. This discussion presents some interventions and options that can be used to provide the corrective experience. The corrective experience is what makes for a group therapeutic factor.

There are numerous interventions and options whose choice will depend on the leader, the needs of a particular member, and the needs of the entire group. This is where a leader's expertise is essential; to select from a wide array of choices and, to be able to select immediately. The impact is greater when the intervention is present centered. Some choices are the following:

- Do nothing.
- Identify the goal of the behavior out loud for the member.
- Meet the need underlying the goal.
- Infuse objective reality.
- Relate behavior and goal to current experiencing and relationships for the member.
- Make a group process comment.

A leader can absorb the information and do nothing. It may not be the best time in the life of the group to make an intervention, the member may not be at a point where they are ready to hear and use the information, or it would be disruptive to something more urgent taking place in the group. *Doing nothing* does not mean ignoring the behavior, goal, or family of origin issues. It is an active choice to do nothing. The member is not punished, denigrated, or shamed for what was said or done. The authority figure did not become angry, upset, sad, blaming and so on.

Another option is to *identify the behavior and goals for the behavior* for the member. Sometimes, just bringing this to someone's attention is sufficient to get them thinking about associations with their possible family of origin issues. Just bringing the behavior and goal to awareness can also be a first step on that road. When members are faced with accepting that this is their behavior and a possible goal, the leader can then begin to help them make associations and direct their focus to family of origin issues.

It could be helpful to that member for the leader to meet the need underlying the goal. For example, if the goal was to gain attention, a leader could provide some attention. This action by the leader could be one of the few times this member was able to get their need met right off the bat. This empathic response is a corrective emotional experience.

Infusing objective reality refers to the leader pointing out possible transference and projections and other members agree what happened and the collective experience was different from what this member responded to or did. Not only was the member's behavior off target it was a clear reflection of previously identified family of origin issues. This intervention would be most helpful if used after a therapeutic relationship was established, and when the member had identified some of their unresolved issues related to family of origin. Using the intervention before these two conditions are in place will probably be counterproductive.

Related to the previous option, but less threatening, is to *associate* the member's behavior and goal in the group *with current experiencing and relationships*. This can be particularly effective when the current relationships mirrors family of origin issues, or there are continuing family relationships that can be highlighted. Beginning with the present can be preliminary to exploring the past. For example, if the member tended to try and rescue others to prevent them from experiencing intense emotions, the leader could describe the behavior, encourage members in the group to respond with their reactions, and connect this to family of origin experiences.

The final choice discussed here is for the leader to make a *group process comment*. This choice would be used when there are considerable commonalties among group members for the behavior and goals. Note that members do not have to have common family-of-origin issues. What is common will be the behaviors and goals. What produces the commentary is the behavior and impact on relationships in the group. Associated with this current experiencing is the family of origin issues that may be different for each member. Group process commentary would identify the seductive, competitive, rivalry, and other such behaviors taking place in the group for all members, not just a few.

Vignette

> *Each group member has reported on family of origin experiences where they repeatedly felt neglected and marginalized in getting their needs met. The reasons ranged from parental emotional abuse, absent parents due to military service or employment, the birth of siblings to maternal depression. The group process comment could be something like this: "Group members are wondering if I and other members are willing to give attention to their needs, and are asking for this in disguised ways, such as being silent, starting disagreements, interrupting each other, challenging me, and so on. It would be more constructive to directly ask for what you want from me and other members."*

Group members may not adjust and change their behavior immediately, but some will try, they will continue to think about the comment and make attempts to ask for what they want. This will be new behavior and may take a while for them to see the value and/or change the years of ingrained behavior. What the comment will do for the group is to give members an opportunity to discuss how their relationships may have been impacted by their indirect assumptions based on family of origin experiences.

References

Ackerman, S. & M. Hilsenroth (2001). A review of therapist characteristics and techniques negatively impacting the therapeutic alliance. *Psychotherapy: Theory, Research, Practice, Training*, 38(2), 171–185.

Agazarian, Y. (1997). *Systems-Centered Therapy for Groups*. New York: Guilford Press.

Andersen, S., & Berk, M. (1998). The social-cognitive model of transference: Experiencing past relationships in the present. *Review of General Psychology*, 2, 81–120.

Beutler, L., Moleiro, C., & Talebi, H. (2002). Resistance in psychotherapy: What conclusions are supported by research. *Journal of Clinical Psychology*, 58(2), 207–217.

Bion, W. (1961). *Experiences in Groups*. New York: Basic Books.

Brown, N. (1998). *The Destructive Narcissistic Pattern*. Westport, CT: Praeger.

Brown, N. (2021). The significance and importance of repairing empathic failures. In Y. I. Kane, S. Masselink, & A. Weiss (Eds.), *Women, Intersectionality and Power in Group Psychotherapy*. New York: Routledge.

Freud, A. (1946). *The Ego and the Mechanisms of Defense*. New York: International Universities Press.

Freud, S. (1953 [1912]). The dynamics of transference. In J. Strachey (Ed.), *The Standard Edition of the Complete Psychological Works of Sigmund Freud*, vol. 12 (pp. 97–108). Richmond: Hogarth Press.

Freud, S. (1936 [1926]). *Inhibitions, Symptoms and Anxiety*. Richmond: Hogarth Press.

Fritscher, L. (2021). How counter-transference can impact your therapeutic relationship. Retrieved from www.verywellmind.com/counter-transference-2671577.

Fueres, J., Gelso, C., Owings, J., & Cheng, D. (2013). Real relationship, wrong alliance, transference and countertransference in time-limited counseling and psychotherapy. *Counselling Psychology Quarterly*, 26(3–4), 294–312.

Hartman, H. (1958). *Ego Psychology and the Problem of Adaptation*. New York: International Universities Press.

Hays, J., Gelso, C., & Hummel, A. (2011). Managing countertransference. *Psychotherapy*, 48(1), 88.

Hays, J., Gelso, C., Goldberg, S., & Kivlighan, D. (2018). Countertransference management and effective psychotherapy: Meta-analytic findings. *Psychotherapy*, 55(4), 496–507.

Hoffer, W. (1952). The mutual influences in the development of ego and id: Earliest stages. *Psychoanalytic Study of the Child*, 7, 31–41.

Kernberg, O. (1990). *Borderline and Narcissistic Conditions*. New York: Aronson.

Leahy, R. (2003). *Overcoming Resistance in Cognitive Therapy*. New York: Guilford Press.

Racker, H. (2018). *Transference and Countertransference*. New York: Routledge.

Reich, W. (1972). *Character Analysis*. New York: Simon & Schuster.

Rosenberg, L., *et al.* (2021). The meaning of together: Exploring Transference and countertransference in palliative care settings. *Journal of Palliative Medicine*, 24, 11.

Thorenson, P. (1972). Defense mechanism in groups. In J. W. Pheiffer & J. E. Jones (Eds.), *The 1971 Annual Handbook for Group Facilitators*. LaJolla CA: University Associates.

11 Virtual and Restricted–Setting Therapy Groups

Introduction

Group therapy made significant changes because of the COVID-19 pandemic, which led to group sessions conducted virtually. These *telegroups* have emerged as a vital force for delivery of group treatment. These groups are valuable for the treatment of a variety of issues, problems and concerns as this modality brings opportunities for a wide variety of people who might not otherwise have access to therapy. It is likely that telegroups will continue to expand and grow.

Telegroups bring benefits and new challenges for the group leader which are addressed in this chapter. Also presented are the importance of pre-planning, technical concerns, modifications of the usual group facilitative group leader sills, and suggestions for implementing and enhancing telegroups.

Telegroups

Let's begin with an activity to bring you into the here and now and focus on the positive aspects of group experiences.

Activity: Group Reflection and Image

Materials: It will be helpful if you can write your responses to the activity and keep it where it is easily assessable when reading subsequent chapters. Paper and a writing instrument are used.

Directions – Sit in a quiet place, close your eyes if you like and visualize a virtual group that you were the leader or a member.

1 Write a short description of the group as you remember it noting the feelings you had then and are now aware of about that group.
2 Now identify and write the most positive experience(s) associated with this group, the most negative experience(s), what you did as the leader or member that was most effective, what you did that was least

DOI: 10.4324/9781003329787-11

effective, what you think or wish that you had done differently as a member or as the leader.

3   Now close your eyes again and form an image of the group and give that image a name or title.

This chapter begins with this activity to better ground you about your feelings and attitudes about groups held virtually and the impacts on the group leader, the group members and the group process. What follows does not address all of the different ways that virtual groups may be held, it is focused on synchronous live video groups (Luxton et al., 2016).

There have been numerous studies on the effectiveness of virtual groups for various issues, conditions and problems and more will be emerging rapidly because of the need to go virtual for the pandemic. Researchers have found favorable outcomes for virtual treatment for panic disorder (Lustgarten, 2017), anxiety (Bischoff et al., 2017), depression (Bischoff et al., 2017), PTSD (Lauckner & Whitten, 2016), military-related combat PTSD (Acierno et al., 2016), substance abuse (Lustgarten, 2017), chronic pain (Lustgarten, 2017), and obsessive-compulsive disorder (Stubbings, Rees, & Roberts, 2015). Studies for different populations have also found favorable results such as juvenile offenders (Batastini et al., 2020), parent training (Comer et al., 2017), refugees with PTSD (Ghumann et al., 2016), at risk for suicide (Gilmore & Ward-Ciesielski, 2017) adolescent depression (Kobak et al., 2015) military with depression (Luxton et al., 2016). What is somewhat lacking in the literature at this time are studies on the effectiveness of group therapy as all of these studies did not use group treatment.

Benefits and Challenges

Benefits for members include increased access to services, the possibilities of feeling less anxious or threatened, decreased emotional contagion, increased ability to be emotionally present in session, fewer missed sessions and/or tardiness, increased ability to attend sessions. Increased access to services includes costs to the member such as transportation and childcare, member availability at designated times is easier, members in rural and other such areas can receive treatment that might not be available in their communities, are definite benefits for the members. This access can also result in fewer missed sessions or being tardy, a reduction in their isolation and alienation, and other positive outcomes. The virtual sessions can also produce less anxiety about their inclusion/exclusion in the group and how they will be perceived by group members. There can also be a reduction in emotional contagion due to the distance and separation of group members, could improve their ability to be and stay emotionally present in sessions and other benefits for members.

There are also some less than positive factors for group members in a virtual setting. They may lack the necessary reliable technology, their space for attending the group may be harder to ensure lack of disruptiveness and intrusions which then reduces privacy and confidentiality as well as what they are willing to disclose technical difficulties that cause frustration during sessions, and other such constraints. In addition, members may experience a lessening of their verbal spontaneity for input and responses, have uncertainty about when to speak, and may find it more difficult to develop a d therapeutic alliance,

Benefits for group leaders include more assurance of members' attendance, the ability to provide treatment and care for remote group members and thus increase their access to care, and it may be easier to structure and direct psychoeducational group sessions (Lopez et al., 2020). In addition, virtual groups can be beneficial for group leaders in that they can more easily provide sessions in settings such as prisons, residential facilities, nursing homes and other venues where access to treatment may be more limited.

Adjusting to a virtual group environment presents many challenges for group leaders in terms of technology requirements, ethical considerations, establishing a therapeutic relationship, constraints for some group factors, and the inability to use some group facilitation strategies and techniques. Among the many difficulties that holding virtual sessions present for group leaders include lost behavioral cues as members move and interact less and only their upper body is visible, it is more difficult to scan the group and note members' reactions, the leader has to look at the camera as part of the better practices for leading virtual groups and this makes it difficult to initiate and maintain eye contact, or to evaluate member's and the group's emotional intensity, the reduction of some therapeutic factors, harder to provide group process comments, establishing the therapeutic alliance, fostering member to member interactions, and a reduction of emotional presence.

Eysenbach et al. (2004) in their review of online groups found that the online groups tended to develop in the same patterns as did in person groups. This pattern of development included the period of becoming acquainted, interacting and setting group norms, and encouraging and supporting group members. They note that groups that had a structured psychoeducational component were more effective than groups organized around a particular condition or problem. Lopez et al. (2020) state that people do find ways to connect in remotely held group settings and are able to interact and connect despite the limitations that these settings present.

Planning and Organizing Telegroup Sessions

Comer et al. (2017) describe the technology requirements and security for virtual sessions that are applicable for virtual group sessions. The technology requirements for both the group leader and members include a computer, camera, microphone, internet connection, and appropriate videoconferencing software. Lustgarten (2017), Luxton et al. (2016), and Swenson et al. (2016) explain that the sessions must be in accord with HIPAA requirements and propose that there be an algorithmic encryption of the video signal to ensure confidentiality. They also state that there should be a backup plan for a technological failure, that the details of the plan should be a part of the written consent, and that it is helpful to have someone with technical expertise on hand to help manage problems.

Much of the success of the virtual group session will rely on the quality of the technology and services such as outdated computers, the reliability and speed of the internet services, and the quality of the audio and video output. When there are continual technical difficulties, computer problems, and/or user inexperience, the leader and group members can become stressed and frustrated. In addition, that means that the focus of the session becomes something other than the designated topic and goal.

Following are some options available for virtual sessions that may be especially helpful for psychoeducational groups; breakout rooms, screen sharing, white board and the chat icon. Breakout rooms can be used to form small groups for discussion. This is especially helpful when the number of group members is greater than 10. This also allows for members to get to know each other in the smaller group and can allow for more expression of thoughts and feelings, as well as promoting interactions among group members. Screen sharing can be done by either the group leader and/or group members. This is where the group leader can share written materials, PowerPoint presentations, handouts for discussions directions for activities and so on. Anything written in advance and saved to a file on the computer can be made visible to group members via this option. The white board option is used for drawing or writing and through screen sharing can be available to both the leader and the designated group members. The chat icon is very helpful for group members and the group leader can ask them to record their thoughts, feelings, and questions for the group and/or for the leader through the chat. Material put under chat is available for viewing by all group members. Lopez et al. (2020) recommend that group leaders use practice sessions to become familiar with the technology as they report that group members are more comfortable when the group leader is familiar and comfortable with using it. They also recommend that group members be offered a practice session.

Another technology-related task is to decide how speaking will be organized so that members can be guided to speak, decrease interruptions, and allow for interactions and discussions. Group members can signal their desire to speak by raising their hand either physically or electronically,

It is recommended that group leaders create their space to be free from distractions, disruptions, or interruptions to include silencing phone and other devices and to have this as a requirement for group members. Pay attention to the background for the leader and try to keep clutter, personal objects and the like either absent or minimal, and a digital background is also a possibility. The attention should be on the group leader, not their background.

Sessions will be less stressful if the leader and group members can reduce background noises as these sounds can give rise to anxieties about confidentiality and privacy, arouse curiosity which distracts from being emotionally present in the session, and some sounds may be alarming to some people. The easiest way to reduce the noises is to have members mute their microphones, but this may not be the best option as the leader will want members to be able to join in at any time. Depending on the level of maturity of the group members they can be requested to mute their microphones until ready to speak, but this then gives some members who already are resistant an excuse for not having input. Members can be requested to do what they can to reduce or eliminate background noises and the location of where they have to be during the session will influence their ability to attend to this.

The group leader should ensure that all needed materials are readily available before starting the session. It is very disruptive to the process when materials and the like have to be secured from another location even if that location is just next door. Forgetting materials or not having enough materials is more easily managed when sessions are in person, but that leader lapse is still disruptive to the process.

Ethics and Professional Issues

Most of the ethical and professional issues that apply in other settings also apply in virtual settings but may have other implications for practice. The basics for these are presented in Chapter 3 and you are encouraged to read your major professional or licensure ethical standards and guidelines. Briefly presented are the major issues and/or constraints for confidentiality, documentation and required reporting, state, and federal ways for working across state lines and scope of practice.

Confidentiality is of importance but cannot be guaranteed and with virtual groups it becomes even more difficult to ensure. Group leaders may find it helpful to state at the beginning of the group the expectation for confidentiality and to also note the constraints and barriers that may exist. For example, some virtual platforms will automatically record sessions unless this feature has to be turned off. Group leaders may not know that the recording option exists unless they seek out the information. There is also the constraint that group members may have that reduces or eliminates confidentiality such as when they do not have a space for their sessions that will be free from interruptions or disruptions by other people. While leaders will want to encourage members' disclosures, they do have to stay mindful that confidentiality may not be ensured.

Documentation and required reporting can be a responsibility for some group leaders such as those who work in courts, agencies, hospitals, and residential settings. This too is something that group leaders should tell group members at the beginning of the group as part of the informed consent especially when this reporting and/or documents are a part of the expectation for the group leader. Leaders are also cautioned to be circumspect in what they write in these reports as well as what is written for personal case notes as the reports and case notes are subject to review by the group member and/or their guardian, can be required with court ordered subpoenas and may be read in open court. A good practice is to write only what you want the group member to read.

State and federal laws for working across state lines have and are changing and it is recommended that group leaders who are working with group members in remote settings stay abreast with the current laws that govern their group work especially of some of the settings are in other states.

Scope of practice is a basic ethical concept in that there may be specialized training needed by group leaders before application to the group. This may be especially true for the use of some techniques such as EMDR, Guided Imagery, and other techniques that have the potential for causing harm if not implemented in accord with that technique's principles. This is why group leaders are encouraged to stay within their scope of practice, and to seek out the specialized training for techniques they want to use.

Managing Group Factors and Group Dynamics

Some group facilitation factors that will need to be managed are building the connections so that trust and safety are established for group members, for the leader to be able to tune in to the group's feeling tone as a cue for what the group may be feeling, encouraging members' expression of their thoughts and feelings, and fostering interactions among group members. Although some studies have shown that establishing a relationship with the leader is easier for group members than it is for them to establish meaningful connections with each other, there are several strategies that may be helpful for group leaders (Lopez et al., 2020).

Tip: Some strategies that may help to build a sense of connections in the group are to encourage members to talk about what is and is not working for them in the virtual group, to identify the losses they are experiencing such as not being able to see some nonverbal cues, and to talk to each other by using their names that are visible on the screen.

While it may be more difficult to tune in to the group's feeling tone and to have members express their feeling.

Tip: Leaders can ask members to identify their feelings either verbally or through the chat icon to get a sense of the general feeling tone of the group.

Asking about feelings may be something that the leader generally uses, and there are points in the sessions or during the duration of the group where this could be a valuable clue for the leader. Some members may not be comfortable with verbalizing their feelings so asking them write these on the chat would be helpful to encourage their feeling expressions.

Tip: Leaders may want to encourage members to use the chat icon during the session to write their thoughts, feelings and ideas or questions as these emerge during the session as this is another means to encourage participation where members may be reluctant to interrupt the members who are speaking or the leader.

Encouraging member-to-member interactions may also be a challenge with virtual group sessions as members may be unfamiliar with group interactions in general but especially so using technology.

Tip: Just as with in person sessions, the leader can ask members to use each other's names to direct their comments and remarks, to talk to each other instead of just to and through the leader, or to even raise their hands, physically or electronically, to talk to each other.

It may take longer for group members to become comfortable with these exchanges and the group leader may have to encourage them to communicate more often.

There are also some group level dynamics that must be attended to and managed in the virtual setting. Among these are group level resistance, conflict, difficult member behaviors, identifying the session's theme, empathic failures and their repairs, and the extent to which the session is present-centered.

Group-level resistance occurs when the group as a whole is avoiding, ignoring, or suppressing something members find to be threatening or dangerous about or in the group at that time. Their apprehensions may be on the unconscious or nonconscious level, and each group member is trying to manage this in their own unique way of resisting. What the group may be fearful of happening is in the group and can be something like open conflict among group members or with the leader, unspoken concerns or dissatisfaction with the leader that may be real or their way of seeking independence from the leader, or the fears can be around intimacy in the group. All of this is much more difficult to identify and manage in the virtual setting but the same strategies that are used in face-to-face group settings can be used here. Group leaders need to be aware of what the group as a whole may be resisting.

Conflict will emerge in group, and this can range from mild disagreements to very intense exchanges. While there are some in person groups that may expect or experience physical violence, this is one of the benefits of virtual groups in that members are in separate spaces so there is less likelihood that physical aggression will result. Tolerance of conflict and working through differences even minor ones can be a valuable teaching tool for psychoeducational groups to illustrate to members how to work through conflicts, the value of trying to resolve minor differences so that they do not become major ones, and that relationships do not have to be destroyed with conflict.

Virtual groups will also have some difficult member behaviors that can negatively affect the group and its progress. Members will bring their usual selves and behaviors to the group regardless of the venue so that if they monopolize in their everyday lives, they will do the same in the group setting. Some of the following suggestions will be helpful for some difficult member behaviors in the virtual settings.

Monopolizing – wait until this is clearly a pattern of behavior and then block at some point. Also add after blocking either a statement about what it would be more helpful to say or do, or what the goal is for that person such as discomfort with silence.

Reflection: What do you use as indicators that a member is monopolizing? It could be helpful to reflect on whether or not the group is supporting this behavior.

Yes – but – give an empathic response as to that member's frustration with not being able to find the solution or answers they think would fit. Ask them what they think would fit their dilemma or problem.

Reflection: Do you find it difficult to not challenge this behavior as the member's resistance to suggestions? If so, it can be helpful to reflect on your desire to provide answers for them and your feelings when none from you or other members are acceptable.

Prolonged silence, withdrawal – Tell the member what was observed that is that they haven't spoken for some time, invite their input, or acknowledge their need for reflection.

Reflection: If this is that member's characteristic behavior does it cause you to feel inept, or that the member is deliberately withholding regardless of the validity of their reason for doing so, or other negative feelings or thoughts? Try to focus more on the possible goal(s) for this behavior and that may give you a clue as to how to effectively bring them into the discussion.

Story-telling – Block the story and ask the member to tell the group what their feelings and thoughts are. Tell them that the details are not important for understanding what is essential and important to them about the topic or event or person.

Reflection: Has this member told the same story several times? If so, having them just focus on their feelings and bring the group members into the discussion can be helpful. Also, consider if the group is allowing this to happen to prevent their having to disclose or the like.

Empathic failures and repairs were addressed in Chapter 5 and are as important for the virtual sessions. It may be harder to note members' feelings about being empathically failed through their nonverbal cues, but the same is true when the session is held face to face as many members tend to hide their reactions. This is one reason why identifying empathic failures and instituting repairs may be of vital importance for virtual sessions.

As noted before, trying to manage group factors and interactions can be a challenge in the virtual setting.

Use of Activities

There are three major considerations for using activities. First, is the choice of type of activity, second is the availability of materials needed for the activity, and the third relates to the first consideration and is the possibility of evoked emotions. Choices of activity are somewhat more limited than for in-person groups, but there are many that will be possible and useful.

Some activities will be more difficult to use in the virtual setting than others. For example, it can be relatively easy to use writing activities, music, and movement activities whereas it is much more difficult to use art-based ones, not impossible, just more difficult. Some of the constraints about using activities include having the materials available, instructions, and time for reporting. Let's review some categories of activities for their ease and difficulty in the virtual environment.

Choice of Activity

Writing activities such as *expressive writing* (Pennebaker, 1997a, 1997b) lists, and brief essays can be easily used. An example of an easily used list activity would be to ask group members to list their strengths. Advantages for using writing activities include that this allows for all group members to participate at the same time around the particular topic, members can be free to choose what they disclose about what they wrote, and the act of writing can help focus their thoughts and feelings. Disadvantages can include the absence of needed materials for a member, their fears about not writing well although this does not matter for these activities, and a reluctance to try and express their thoughts and feelings in this way.

Music activities (Brown, 2013) can be used to energize, to calm, or to evoke emotions but not for deeper explorations such as those used by music therapists. It is important that the group leader has an understanding of what may be evoked by their selection of particular pieces of music as well as knowing a wide range of types of music that can be employed. Advantages of using music can be to soothe, calm, relieve tension, promote feelings of well-being, energize, and the like. Disadvantages are that the type of music selected may not be pleasing for all group members and that some pieces may evoke unintended distressing memories. In fact, there can be some types of music that are distasteful for some people.

Art-based activities require the availability of art materials such as crayons, felt markers, colored pencils, paint, pens or pencils for drawing activities and glue sticks, scissors, colored paper, and other such materials for collages. When groups meet face to face it was recommended that the group leader provide these materials, but this cannot be easily done when the group meets virtually, and group leaders usually have to ask group members to get the needed materials. Not supplying members with the materials can result in their not having the materials for an activity when needed for a variety of reasons. That usually leads to frustration on both the leader and members' parts as the activity cannot be implemented unless all members have the materials. This is one reason why the choice of activity is so important, and it is difficult to use art-based activities in the virtual space. The biggest constraint may be member's resistance to anything art-based because of the erroneous idea that the activities require artistic talent, and this can be more difficult to overcome in the virtual setting.

Movement activities may be more difficult to implement due to space concerns. Examples of movement activities are dance, yoga, stretching, or even running in place. The intent of movement is to use the body as a means to access feelings, experience different bodily sensations, relax, or energize. However, space is needed for moving around and this may be limited for both the leader and group members.

Availability of Materials

There are numerous activities that are useful for psychoeducational groups, but these can be difficult to implement in the virtual setting because of the availability of materials such as with art-based activities. The biggest constraint will be members' access to needed materials. Usually these are supplied by the group leader for a particular activity and the leader secures the materials needed for the activity in advance of implementation. Another constraint is the cost of materials. While some materials may be of little cost, having to have a variety of these can start to add up and become expensive. Also, group members may not have access to places that stock low-cost art materials.

Evoked Emotions

There is always the possibility of evoking emotions for members when using activities and some activities and that can be the purpose for some activities. There are times when the evoked emotion can be distressful and/or intense and group leaders must stay mindful and aware of this possibility which is even more important for virtual leadership. Members do not always speak of the distressful evoked emotion and when the session is face to face, it can be easier for the group leader to recognize when a member is distress or some other reactions for an evoked emotion. Some visual cues are definitely missing or more easily hidden with virtual sessions. Leaders can make it a part of the expansion phase to ask members to verbalize evoked emotions.

Orientation Session

Plan to have an orientation session either before the group begins or as an integral part of the first session. The orientation should include group rules and expectations and the technical aspects of virtual sessions.

While members may have had experience with other types of groups, it can reduce some of their anxiety about the ambiguity and uncertainty around this particular group experience to present some information about the rules of the group and expectations of members. It is most helpful if the group leader can prepare these in advance and to have them in writing so that they can be sent to group members such as via email. Suggested basic group rules would include the following:

- Attend all session and arrive on time.
- Notify the group leader when sessions will be missed.
- Attend sessions where there are no distractions, disruptions, and the like to maintain confidentiality for group members.
- Actively participate.

Some group members may not be familiar with technology and can find that their participation is affected because of this lack of information. This is why the orientation session is best held before the group begins. Members can be told what the session will cover and can elect to be absent if they do not need the information. Technical aspects that can be a part of the virtual sessions and helpful to cover in the orientation include muting, how to be recognized, how and when to use the chat function, and sharing screen.

Group leaders may want to have group members mute their micro-phones when not speaking so that any background noises will be elimi-nated. However, it is best to ask members to keep their videos on all of the time and not to black them out during the session.

Options for when members want to provide input, disclose ask or answer a question or when and how to speak include using the raise hand function on zoom, physically raising the hand so that it is seen on camera, and using the zoom chat function. The group leader can use all of these and tell members about the options during the orientation. Use of the chat function can also allow members to provide responses to the group member who is speaking as well as using it in other ways such as to provide their input. The group leader who wants to use this chat function will need to have some guidelines for how it may be used, and to also monitor the postings during the sessions.

Some groups such as psychoeducational groups have dissemination of information as one of its methods and the Zoom *share screen* function is useful for this. It is also possible to use the function to allow group members to write and present information, thoughts, and the like. During orientation, the group leader can explain what share screen is and how it will be used in the group.

Cues for Virtual Sessions

Although many of the usual cues are not available for virtual sessions, there are some nonverbal communication cues that will be helpful for group leaders to look for and attend to. Among these are facial expressions, voice tone, and upper body gestures.

Notice facial expressions especially when there are changes and shifts. Cues can be discerned from the eye movements, presence or absence of smiles, and noticing the general impression of the facial expression. Some information can be gleaned from the overall impression the group leader receives when looking at the member's face.

Voice tones can be revealing of the person's emotional state. For example, when someone talks fast, choppy, and loud, that can be an indication of some emotional intensity about the topic or disclosure. Notice when group members' voice tones change during the session, are different in a particular session and what impression or reaction is provoked in the group leader. This can be cues for suppression of feelings especially intense negative feelings which can then lead to more effective interventions.

Although the entire body is not usually seen on the computer screen, there are some cues to what members may be experiencing at that moment from the positions and/or movement of their heads, shoulders, hand gestures, and/or head positions. This is why it can be helpful for the group leader to attend to how the member is physically presenting themself on the computer screen.

Discussion/reflection: Identify how therapeutic ruptures could emerge in a Telegroup and how the leader could intervene and repair these. Do the same for microaggressions.

Restricted Group Environments

There are some settings where the rules and regulations will set a restricted group environment and these will affect the type of group, leadership tasks, actions, and the like for the leader and for group members. Examples for restricted group settings include inpatients in hospitals, outpatient, residential care, agencies, prisons, and schools for examples. The extent of the restrictions will depend on the type of organization and its mission. Examples for missions are usually treatment, rehabilitation and for prisons, punishment. Brabender & Fallon (2019) note that the mission and theoretical orientation of the organization provide the framework for the groups that will be conducted. Essential when planning groups for these restricted environments are program elements such as treatment, interactions and input from other program elements, specific restrictions that impact the group and its members, and the like. It is recommended that group leaders try to fully understand what the organizational goals for group therapy are, how ethical concerns are addressed such as confidentiality, documentation, and reporting requirements, prior to the start of the group. The differences among and between facilities that may be restricted are too numerous to try and address here. The focus will be to identify the major considerations for group leaders.

Leader Concerns

The major concerns for group leaders working in restricted environments are their limited authority, selection of group members, ethical concerns such as reporting and documentation, and limitations on use of activities.

The group leader in restricted environments may have *limited authority* to make some decisions as the organization may have set these in advance. For example, structural components such as the number and/or length of sessions, the size of the group, if the group is open or closed, the location for the group sessions, theoretical perspective and if there is a co-leader may be predetermined by the organization. It is unlikely that the leader will be able to *screen members* for their suitability for the group nor the authority to prevent them from attending. *Ethical concerns* include to do no harm, informed consent, duty to warn/protect, reporting and documentation, and interactions with other professionals in the setting.

Some Constraints

Each setting will differ in the constraints that will affect the leader, the group and the members. Examples of some major constraints are the composition of the group, outside group interactions, and use of materials for activities. The setting will determine the composition of the group and leaders it is possible that members for a particular group can vary widely in age, educational level, extent of support systems, and so on. While it is likely also that groups will be composed of peers, for some treatment and rehabilitation organizations may have significant differences among clients. Another constraint may be an expectation that members will have outside of the group interactions where they can and will discuss group topics, disclosures, and other sensitive materials. For example, in a residential center group members are living in proximity to each other and engaging in other communal activities. Prevention of discussions for group topics and the like may be impossible to expect. The final major constraint presented here is the use of materials for activities that may be prohibited. There are many settings such as schools and residential where the participants are prohibited from using anything that may be used as a potential weapon such as scissors, pencils, or even glue. Leaders are advised to check with the authorities at the setting about what materials and activities may be used for group.

It can be helpful for group leaders to consult the literature about the diagnosis(es) for the group members to better understand their symptoms, treatment possibilities, and a guide for containing their behavior, thoughts, and feelings. Consultation with the professionals at the setting can also be of help to better plan the group sessions, and to understand what takes place between group sessions. The final suggestion is that leaders develop a realistic expectation for the interactions in sessions and the outcomes of groups held in restricted settings.

References

Acierno, R. D., *et al.* (2016). Behavioral activation and therapeutic exposure for posttraumatic stress disorder: A noninferiority trial of treatment delivered in person versus home-based telehealth. *Depression and Anxiety*, 33(5), 415–423. doi:10.1002/da.22476.

Batastini, A., *et al.* (2020). Are videoconferenced mental and behavioral health services just as good as in-person? A meta-analysis of a fast growing practice. *Clinical Psychology Review*. doi:10:1016/j.cpe.2020.101944.

Bischoff, R., Springer, P., & Taylor, N. (2017). Global mental health in action: Reducing disparities one community at a time. *Journal of Marital and Family Therapy*, 43(2), 276–290.

Brabender, V., & Fallon, A. (2019). *Group Psychotherapy in Inpatient, Partial Hospital, and Residential Care Settings*. Washington, DC: American Psychological Association.

Braeuer, K., Noble, N., & Yi, S. (2022). The efficacy of an online anger management program for justice-involved youth. *Journal of Addictions & Offender Counseling*, 43(1), 26–37. doi:10.1002/jaoc.12101.

Brown, N. (2013). *Creative Activities for Group Therapy*. New York: Routledge.

Burlingame, G, McClendon, D. & Alonso, J. (2011). Cohesion in group therapy. *Psychotherapy*, 48, 34–42. doi:10.1037/a00222063.

Catroppa, C., *et al.* (2021). Evaluating the feasibility and efficacy of the Amsterdam memory and attention training for children (Amat-c) following acquired brain injury (ABI): Protocol for a pilot study with online clinician support. *Brain Impairment*, 23(3). doi:10.1017/BrImp.2021.13.

Comer, J. J., *et al.* (2017). Remotely delivering real-time parent training to the home: An initial randomized of internet delivered Parent-Child Interaction Therapy (I-PCIT). *Journal of Consulting and Clinical Psychology*, 85(8), 831–834. doi:10.1037/ccp0000230.

Eysenbach, G., *et al.* (2004). Health related virtual communities and electronic support groups: systematic review of the effects of online peer to peer interactions. *BMJ*, 328, 1166. doi:10.1136/bmj.328.7449.1166.

Frohlich, J. R., *et al.* (2021). Efficacy of a minimally guided internet treatment for alcohol misuse and emotional problems in young adults: Results of a randomized controlled trial. *Addictive Behaviors Reports*, 14, 100390. doi:10.1016/j.abrep.2021.100390.

Gentry, M., Lapid, M., Clark, M., & Rummans, T. (2018). Evidence for telehealth group-based treatment: A systematic review. *Journal of Telemedicine and Telecare*, 25(6), 327–342.

Ghumman, U., McCord, C., & Chang, J. (2016). Posttraumatic stress disorder in Syrian refugees: A review. *Canadian Psychology*, 57(4), 246–253.

Gilmore, A., & Ward-Ciesielski, E. (2017). Perceived risks and use of psychotherapy via telemedicine for patients at risk for suicide. *Journal of Telemedicine and Telecare*, 25(1). doi:10.1177/1357633X17735559.

Hepburn, K., Nocera, J., Higgins, M., Epps, F., Brewster, G. S., Lindauer, A., Morhardt, D., Shah, R., Bonds, K., Nash, R., & Griffiths, P. C. (2021). Results of a randomized trial testing the efficacy of Tele-Savvy, an online synchronous/asynchronous psychoeducation program for family caregivers of persons living with dementia. *The Gerontologist*, 62(4), 616–628. doi:10.1093/geront/gnab029.

Karagiozi, K., Margaritidou, P., Tsatali, M., Marina, M., Dimitriou, T., Apostolidis, H., Tsiatsos, T., & Tsolaki, M. (2021). Comparison of on site versus online psycho education groups and reducing caregiver burden. *Clinical Gerontologist*, 45 (5), 1330–1340. doi:10.1080/07317115.2021.1940409.

Kobak, K., Mundt, J., & Kennar, B. (2015). Integrating technology into cognitive behavior therapy for adolescent depression: A pilot study. *Annals of General Psychiatry*, 14, 37–47. doi:10.1186/s12991-015-0077-8.

Lauckner, C., & Whitten, P. (2016). The state and sustainability of telepsychiatry programs. *Journal of Behavioral Health Services & Research*, 43(2), 305–318. doi:10:1007/s11414-015-9461-z.

Lopez, A., Rothberg, B., Reaser, E., Schwenk, S., & Griffin, R. (2020). Therapeutic groups via video teleconferencing and the impact on group cohesion. *MHealth*, 6, 13. doi:10.21037/mhealth.2019.11.04.

Lustgarten, S. (2017). Ethical concern for telemental health therapy amidst governmental surveillance, *American Psychologist*, 72(2), 159–170. doi:10.1037/a0040321.

Luxton, D. L., *et al.* (2016). Home-based telebehavioral health for U.S. military personnel and veterans with depression: A randomized controlled trial. *Journal of Consulting and Clinical Psychology*, 84(11), 923–934. doi:10.1037/ccp0000135.

Meyer, K., Glassner, A., Norman, R., James, D., Sculley, R., LealVasquez, L., Hepburn, K., Liu, J., & White, C. (2022). Caregiver self-efficacy improves following complex care training: Results from the Learning Skills Together pilot study. *Geriatric Nursing*, 45, 147–152. doi:10.1016/j.gerinurse.2022.03.013.

Naini, R., Wibowo, M. E., & Mulawarman, M. (2021). Efficacy of online group counseling with mindfulness-based cognitive approach to enhance students' humility. *Islamic Guidance and Counseling Journal*, 4(1), 78–90. doi:10.25217/igcj. v4i1.1280.

Northover, C., Deacon, J., King, J., & Irons, C. (2021). Developing self-compassion online: Assessing the efficacy and feasibility of a brief online intervention. *OBM Integrative and Complementary Medicine*, 6(4), 1–1. doi:10.21926/obm. icm.2104056.

Pang, Y., Zhang, X., Gao, R., Xu, L., Shen, M., Shi, H., Li, Y., & Li, F. (2021). Efficacy of web-based self-management interventions for depressive symptoms: a meta-analysis of randomized controlled trials. *BMC Psychiatry*, 21(1). doi:10.1186/s12888-021-03396-8.

Pennebaker, J. W. (1997a). *Opening Up: The Healing Power of Expressing Emotion.* New York: Guilford.

Pennebaker, J. W. (1997b). Writing about emotional experiences as a therapeutic process. *Psychological Science*, 8, 162–166.

Rentala, S. (2021). Efficacy of psychoeducation to improve medication adherence among bipolar affective disorder: A systematic review. *Indian Journal of Psychiatric Nursing*, 18(1), 55.

Stubbings, D., Rees, C., & Roberts, L. (2015). New avenues to facilitate engagement in psychotherapy: The use of videoconferencing and text-chat in a severe case of obsessive-compulsive disorder. *Australian Psychologist*, 50(4), 265–270. doi:10.1111/ap.12111.

Swenson, J., Smothermon, J., Rosenblad, S., & Chalmers, B. (2016). The future is here: Ethical practices of telemental health. *Journal of Psychology and Christianity*, 35(4), 310–319.

Weinberg, H. (2021). Obstacles, Challenges and Benefits of Online Group Psychotherapy. *American Journal of Psychotherapy*, 74(2), 83–88.

Weinberg, H. (2020). Online group psychotherapy: Challenges and possibilities during COVID-19 – A practice review. *Group Dynamics: Theory, Research, and Practice*, 24(3), 201–211.

12 Emerging Group Therapy Concerns and Possibilities

Cybersecurity for Instruction and for Therapists

The precautions presented here are intended for digital devices in common use at this time by instructors and their students, therapists and therapists in training, and their clients. Devices include cell phones, computers, tablets, or any other device that is used to communicate, and/or store, and/or access information. Care should be taken to prevent unintentional theft and other loss, unauthorized access, and other breaches of devices that will put students or clients at risk for intrusions into their privacy and confidential matters, and/or subject them to the same risks as does social media. Discussed are some actions that can help strengthen and secure devices that carry or have access to sensitive information, actions that leave the devices open to unauthorized access, actions that should not be used, and suggestions for uses for therapy. Special attention is given to passwords/passphrases.

Devices can be made more secure with use of the following.

- Auto-lock with a strong password to unlock.
- Keep devices in a secure location.
- Use multifactor authentications.
- Enabling auto-updates, anti-malware, or antivirus.
- Use inactivity loci-out or password protected saver and host-based firewall for laptops and workstations.
- Only use software from reliable sources and use on all devices.
- Disable the guest account and routinely work using a user account.
- Enable erase after a number of unsuccessful login attempts, find-my-device, and remote wipe.

Passwords/passphrases can provide protection to access to devices when certain steps are taken or certain actions are avoided.

- Multiple devices and multiple sites should have different passwords/passphrases. Maybe construct a list for each device in a notebook that is kept in a secure place.

DOI: 10.4324/9781003329787-12

- Strong passwords/passphrases should be created to resist easy guesses and changed often such as every 6 months.
- Do not use the same password/phrase for different sensitive sites, nor store these on your computer or phone.
- Do not use personal or professional passwords/passphrases on public computers as these may be accessed by unauthorized people.
- Change passwords/passphrases whenever there is a security concern.

Data protection includes preventing disclosure of any information that may identify students or clients and/or their sensitive and/or private information. Examples of data that may need protection include but are not limited to emails, therapy notes, reports, grades, addresses, and the like. There are two actions that will help to protect data, encryption, and back-up. Ensure that electronic communications such as emails, reports, scheduling, billing, and payments are encrypted. Ensure that scheduling software is encrypted and secure. Clients and students should be informed of potential risks for transmitting their personal information and data such as grades or a diagnosis. Back-up data often and to a secure location. It is also helpful to verify that websites are encrypted (showing a locked lock image) before submitting a password/passphrase or any sensitive data to the website.

It is essential to stay aware of *connections* such as the internet to access or review sensitive data such as therapy notes, or to open emails, or to deliver telemental health therapy. Suggested is to use a VPN when using a public WiFi network, and to turn off connection services when they are not being used such as Bluetooth, VPN or Location Services.

Therapy Uses

The following are especially useful for therapy.

1   Keep records accessible and secure, back up client files to a secure cloud space and do not store records on your computer as these may be lost with a technical glitch. However you choose to back up files and store records, it is best not to rely solely on electronic devices.
2   HIPPA rules require that sensitive data be encrypted. It is essential that the group leader only communicate with clients using secure encrypted channels and to be especially mindful of email communications since most email will not be automatically encrypted.
3   As part of the telegroup orientation group leaders should read and disseminate the platform's rules and policies. Important for group members to know will be the platform's (such as Zoom) privacy policy, their data collection policies and procedures and other such policies.
4   It can be helpful for group leaders to control who can attend meetings by having a password for sessions and an admittance procedure. Group

leaders should tell members if the sessions are recorded and the process for them accessing their personal information. When sessions are recorded it is best to encrypt them before archiving, to use the best encryption software available.

Cybersecurity incidents are best handled by a cybersecurity expert. Cybersecurity incidents are numerous, and all devices can be subject to these incidents. Examples of incidents include data breaches, ransomware, malware, phishing, unauthorized access to data, unauthorized changes to data or systems, loss or theft of devices or data, a denial of service attack, compromised user accounts, and improper disclosures accidently or because they were left unprotected. Finally, a common incident is the improper disposal of hard drives, USB drives, DVDS, CDs, servers, printers, copiers, or any device that stores information such as a cell phone.

Artificial Intelligence for Instruction

The educational applications for artificial intelligence (AI) are rapidly expanding and evolving, and there are many classroom applications. Artificial Intelligence has been in use for a long time but new developments are causing a deeper thought about its advantages and disadvantages for learning and teaching. This brief discussion is focused on applications of AI for teaching and training specifically for group psychotherapy. Topics included are a definition of AI and an example, possible advantages, disadvantages, examples for instructional applications, and a guide for how instructors can promote their students' professional uses and responsibilities.

AI as an assistant uses data mining to produce answers to prompts or questions. AI has been in use for some time, as evidenced by the use of Siri and Alexa and facial recognition. In short, AI has a specific task to complete and can do that very rapidly. An example of AI used in higher education is that some universities are using it to compute complex analytics such as enrollment analytics, that track prospective students' interest by their interactions with the university's website, their social media posts, and emails. The information derived from these analytics are then used to determine which students to reach out to, what aspects of campus life appeals to them, and even to assess applications. The last application is becoming less trustworthy as prospective students are using AI to write admissions essays that are acceptable and the AI assistance cannot be detected.

Possible advantages for instructors' uses for AI as a writing assistant include but are not limited to drafting emails, writing blogs, cover letters, article summaries, constructing tests and quizzes, and developing discussion questions and topics. AI is shown to be helpful to create course syllabi, and can even assist with composing lectures. There are many positive uses for AI in the classroom that instructors can use for the benefit of students such as AI for editing, setting up AI assisted tutoring, and modifications for assignments.

Possible disadvantages some of which may not be detectable are that the information AI mines may be biased as AI retains all input including biased input which then factors into the output. Also, because AI cannot discriminate between valid and invalid sources, there can be many inaccuracies in its output including factual errors, incomplete quotes, and even erroneous findings. Then there is the important undetermined answer to the ownership of the intellectual property AI develops from a prompt. The professional and legal challenges have yet to be addressed.

There are other major disadvantages because of the difficulties that AI can present for instructors who must evaluate student learning under the conditions presented by AI among which are ethical use, fraud, plagiarism and professional responsibility. Fraud is a difficulty because there are no reliable ways to detect AI work or AI-assisted work for written material. Thus, the instructor will have difficulty in determining if the submitted work is that of the student or if it was assisted by AI or if it is entirely AI work.

Students may not be in the habit of citing sources and this is another difficulty. While the student may not have a conscious intent to plagiarize, they may not know that all sources should be cited for submitted assignments. Instructors may need to be intentional about notifying students who use AI assistance if it is permitted for the class, and most of all that it be cited.

Guide for Instructors

Following are some basic tips for instructors.

- Learn the basics about use of AI for instruction.
- Update course policies to specifically address the use of AI whether it is forbidden, can be partially used and for what, or if it is allowable.
- Review the course assignments to determine how to use or forbid the use of AI.
- Put the course policy for use of AI on the syllabus including penalties if any. Also address the instructor's policy about plagiarism, cheating and note where and how students may use AI for coursework if this is allowed. Give examples of where AI cannot be used relative to the course such as to practice concepts and skills, or where is cannot be used such as for observations that are written for supervision, reports and the like.
- Talk with the students about professional and responsible use and limitation for use of AI for the particular course. If AI or AI assistance is allowed, note the number of points or other credits with as statement such as number of points given for use of submissions using ChatGPT (or other AI).

Ideas for Using AI for Instruction

Constructive AI instructional *uses* for instructors includes the following.

- Develop writing prompts and other activities that will encourage creative thought.
- Develop prompts that can be used by AI to clarify, expand, and/or provide nuances.
- Require students to provide a list of sources consulted, a bibliography and/or citations for written work.
- Assigning students to provide short summaries of group therapy related topics using AI.
- Assign students to use AI to respond to group therapy situations, and then to critique the AI responses.

Examples for student responses to situations

Directions: Provide an intervention for the described group situations.

1 Assume that you are the group leader.
2 The members of the group are similar to students in the class.
3 Your proposed intervention must be implemented in the group session. The intervention may not include taking a member aside or meeting with them outside of the group.
4 The intervention proposed must be consistent with text(s) materials.
5 Assume the situation arises in the fourth or fifth session after the group is under way.

Situation 1

The group does not seem to be able to settle on a topic. The discussion keeps ranging on many out of the group topics and issues. Members seem to be content to just chit chat. How would you intervene as the group leader.

Situation 2

Rudy was an active participant in the previous session until Mary challenged him for taking up so much time. Other group members did not say anything, and Rudy apologized for talking so much. It is now the next session and Rudy has been noticeably quiet this session. All attempts by you and members to solicit his input has failed.

Artificial Intelligence for Psychotherapy

There are numerous studies that have been conducted on the use of Artificial Intelligence (AI) for psychotherapy and more are emerging every day. This presentation is limited to a short description for some AI applications, the advantages and disadvantages for AI for therapy, and a short overview of some studies.

Some frequently used AI applications include chatbots, conversational AI, and embodied AI. *Chatbots* are used for specific roles or to review the interactions between clients and conversational AI. Miner et al. (2018) describes three methods for using AI to augment or replace traditional therapy; AI delivered under human supervision, as an adjunct to traditional therapy with a human, and therapy by AI only. Their examples of how the AI system could be used include the AI offering a call to 911 if a client mentions self-harm in their interaction, and a chatbot can provide a reflective or empathic response. While none of these take the place of a human, it could be that the encouragement and/or support that the chatbot could provide is helpful for some clients.

Conversational AI is defined as the interaction between humans and computers or machines. There are speech enabled applications that will allow a conversation to occur, automated messages such as reminders and check-ins, and other such applications.

Embodied AI includes wearable robots for rehabilitation, robot manufacturing and empathic robots. An example from the literature is the use of embodied robots to care for dementia patients, to gather data and refine treatment plans, and to respond with reflective or empathic responses.

Advantages for using AI in psychotherapy include increased personalized care, shorter wait times, removal of barriers, boost efficiency, helps with monitoring. Conversational AI could be especially helpful with automated messages, use of a speech-based app, and other speech-enabled applications for clients who may not have access to devices for writing or have low writing skills to explain their concerns.

Disadvantages for AI uses are primarily ethical and legal. Of major concern are clients' privacy, informed consent, the risk of surveillance and of obtaining sensitive information about the client, some data that is mined with AI has been shown to be biased, discriminatory, inaccurate and misleading. Some of the same legal concerns relative to the use of social media may also apply to AI with psychotherapy such as stalking, harassment and bullying if client's data is accessed.

Instructors and therapists are advised to stay as current as possible regarding the advances of AI, and also the need to take steps to maintain security, confidentiality and privacy.

Here is list of some sample studies on the uses of AI for psychotherapy since 2018 that include clinical trials, randomized studies, systematic reviews, and other robust methodologies. Results show benefits for addictions (Budney et al., 2019), autism (Burke et al., 2018), acrophobia, emotional problems (Gual-Montolio et al., 2022), psychosis (Craig et al. 2018; de Pierrefeu et al., 2018), depression and anxiety (Fitzpatrick et al, 2017; Fulmer et al., 2018), lung cancer (Liu et al., 2018), life skills (Gabrielli et al., 2020), students (Dekker et al., 2020), and suicide prevention (Rein et al. 2018). This list is not exhaustive and only gives some indices of the current possible uses for AI in psychotherapy.

Social Media for Instruction and Therapy

Social media continues to evolve and often perceived as a viable way to connect to students, engage them, and by extension contribute to their learning, but is not recommended for instruction for group therapy leaders. It is highly recommended that instructors use university approved platforms for teaching purposes. The rationale for the recommendation is presented later in this section, and some of the material in Chapter 11 on virtual teaching and telegroups also applies. Discussed are some of the advantages and teaching possibilities for using social media, the disadvantages, and lastly, some recommended safeguards to implement if used.

Advantages and Disadvantages

Both the advantages and the disadvantages for using social media in therapy are significantly related to ethical and professional concerns (Baier, 2018; Lehanot et al., 2010; Kaplan et al., 2011; Kapoor et al., 2018) and must be carefully considered by the instructor for instruction and the by the group leader for group therapy. In addition, it will be helpful to consult the professional ethical codes for guidance.

Advantages include the instructional media for engaging students such notifications, lecturers, discussions, photo essays, blogs and other such assignments. There are many instructional strategies that can be implemented via social media and some are described in more detained in the section on examples. However, it should also be noted that all of these and others are usually provided by the university's approved platform and instructors are encouraged to use that mechanism for teaching group therapy.

Disadvantages include the following some of which are potentially harmful to students and/or can raise legal concerns in some instances.

- Cyberbullying/trolling defined as sending, posting, or sharing negative, harmful, false or mean content about a person. It can include sharing personal or private information about someone that will cause embarrassment, shame, or humiliation. Some posts may be unlawful or criminal.
- Posting inappropriate content such as opinions unrelated to the course content, pornography, and the like can occur and the instructor cannot prevent this from happening.

- Identity theft can occur especially if there is a requirement to post personal information, or even just knowledge about who is enrolled in the course.
- Privacy concerns are paramount as students may be unaware that by participating they relinquish some privacy that cannot be assured will not be available to others who are not enrolled in the class.
- Authentication of announcements and other postings, participation, materials, and the like cannot be verified as being authentic.
- False information can be posted and even made to appear that it is coming from someone else.
- There is usually no informed consent for student participation in social media for instruction. Students may not be given an alternative and must participate.
- Possible legal concerns related to confidentiality and privacy may emerge.

When non-university licensed platforms are used for instruction there can be concerns about privacy, accessibility, and confidentiality some of which risk conflicting with or violating FERPA. FERPA protects student information such as class enrollment, grades, schedule, location, and other private information. When social media is required for the course that provide opportunities to reveal students' enrollment and participation, comments or feedback could disclose a student grade, class activity planning such as field trips could disclose a student's schedule or location, each of which places the student, the instructor, and the University at risk. In addition, students using social media platforms are disclosing their private information and are providing data feeds for social media data mining engines.

Safeguards can be implemented although they are not fail-safe. The instructor can investigate the platform to determine how the platforms ensures the credibility and accuracy of the information on that platform, the terms of service, whether the platform owns the data generated by the students and/or instructor, and if the creations of the student and/or instructor are copyrighted.

If used, the instructor can take care to do the following.

- Notify students that the platform will be used and the instructional goal. Describe the educational intent and value for using social media.
- Obtain student informed consent before the class begins by developing a form similar to that used for research studies. The informed consent includes the rationale and purpose for using the social media platform, what course units or assignments students will be required to complete or submit via the platform, and the what is needed to access the platform needs. The form should be signed and returned prior to the start of the class.

- Provide alternative options for students unwilling to use social media or who lack accessibility to the platform for example, how assignments can be submitted.
- Establish a password-protected environment that is only accessible by students registered for their class. This should also apply to teaching assistants.
- Institute means to help students stay anonymous such as using a pseudonym or alias.
- Provide a clear statement on the course syllabus that includes the need for software or creating an account on the platform that requires them to use their real name or if a pseudonym can be used.
- Notifications – such as due dates for assignments, unanticipated events affecting the instructor that will affect the class, changes for assignments and the like.

Examples for Constructive Use of Social Media for Instruction

Presented are some examples for instructional use of social media. It should be noted that all of these examples will most likely be available on the university's instructional platform.

- *Lectures* – Instructors can record and posted to be viewed at the students' convenience.
- *Discussions* – Topics can be assigned to discussion to class groups and recorded for the instructor and other students to observe and/or evaluate.
- *Photo essays* –Students are assigned topic(s) for producing an essay using photographs. Topics such as an introduction of oneself, major interests, how to complete a task, and the like can be posted where the instructor and other students can view and provide feedback.
- *Class or individual student blogs* – The instructor can post blogs on course related topics. Course related topics are assigned to students for them to write and post a blog. Blogs can be weekly, or for any time-frame. Instructors can use the blog assignment with or without provisions for comments and questions from the instructor or other students.
- *Crisis strategy* –Instructors can provide a process and/or procedure for individual, group or university crises.
- Groups can be formed such as interest based and/or class assigned groups. These can meet, compare notes, work on projects and the like via social media.
- Students can be assigned YouTube presentation to view and write a review as it relates to or can be applied to class-related topics.

Social Media in Therapy

With the proper safeguards in place, many of the same uses for using social media for instruction are applicable to therapy if the structure for the therapy permits outside of the group interactions. The last point can be the most troubling in that some group members may be too emotionally fragile for these interactions, some may use social media to exploit or bully other group members, unintentional personal information may be disclosed but not shared for all group members thereby producing secrets and a clique, the possibility of "ghosting" and trolling can emerge, and privacy and confidentiality can be compromised depending on the internet connection and/or where it is accessed. The group leader will have no control over how or when social media will be used by group members.

On the other hand, some positive outcomes can be possible such as the following:

- Provide additional support and encouragement.
- Reduce alienation and isolation for some members.
- Track members' progress toward their goals.
- Check-ups and check-ins can be used.
- Activities can be shared such as mindfulness.
- Resources and other information can be shared.
- The group leader can provide individual member coaching.
- Members can share their creative expressions such as art, collages, poetry, and the like.

The challenge for group leaders who choose to use social media for therapeutic purposes will be to balance the possible negative outcomes such as unintentional disclosures with the possible negative outcomes. Interactions between individual and groups of members and the like that take place outside of the group should be brought back to the group so that all group members are aware of them. Leaders will also have to be aware that all group members are not having the same group experience and stay mindful of what the impact of that is on members and on the group.

Summary

Technology is evolving rapidly and the many uses for teaching and for therapy are just beginning to emerge. It is essential that group therapists and their instructors and trainers stay aware of these new advances and how they may be beneficial as well as their possible disadvantages.

References

Baier, A. (2018). The ethical implications of social media: Issues and recommendations for clinical practice. *Ethics and Behavior*, 29(5), 341–351. doi:10.1080/10508422.2018.1516148.

Budney, A., Borodovshy, J., Marsch, L., & Lord, S. (2019). Technological innovations in addiction treatment. In I. Danovitch & L. Mooney (Eds.), *The Assessment and Treatment of Addiction* (pp. 75–90). St. Louis, MO: Elsevier.

Burke, L., et al. (2018). Using virtual interactive training agents (ViTA) with adults with autism and other developmental disabilities. *Journal of Autism Developmental Disorders*, 48, 905–912. doi:10.1007/s10803-017-3374-z.

Craig, T., et al. (2018). AVATAR therapy for auditory verbal hallucinations in people with psychosis: a single-blind, randomized controlled trial. *Lancet Psychiatry* 5, 31–40. doi:10.1016/S2215-0366(17)30427-3.

de Pierrefeu, A., et al. (2018). Prediction of activation patterns preceding hallucinations in patients with schizophrenia using machine learning with structured sparsity. *Hum. Brain Mapp.*, 39, 1777–1788. doi:10.1002/hbm.23953.

Dekker, I., et al. (2020). Optimizing students' mental health and academic performance: AI-enhanced life crafting. *Frontiers of Psychology*, 11, 1063. doi:10.3389/fpsyg.2020.0163.

Fiske, A., Henningsen, P., & Buyx, A. (2019). Your robot therapist will see you now: Ethical implications of embodied artificial intelligence in psychiatry, psychology, and psychotherapy. *Journal of Medical Internet Research*, 2, 1Le13216. doi:10.2196/13216.

Fitzpatrick, K., Darcey, A., & Vierhile, M. (2017). Delivering cognitive behavior therapy to young adults with symptoms of depression and anxiety using a fully automated conversational agent (Woebot): A randomized control trial. *JMIR Journal of Mental Health*, 4, e10. doi:10.2196/mental.7785.

Fulmer, R., et al. (2018). Using psychological artificial intelligence (Tess) to relieve symptoms of depression and anxiety: randomized control trial. *JMIR Mental Health*, 5, e64. doi:10.2196/mental.9782.

Gabrielli, S., Rizzi, S., Carbone, S., & Donisi, V. (2020). A chatbot-based coaching intervention for adolescents to promote life skills: pilot study. *JMIR Human Factors*, 7, e16762. doi:10.2196/16762.

Gual-Montolio, P., et al. (2022). Using AI to enhance ongoing psychological interventions for emotional problems in real or close to real-time: A systematic review. *Environmental Research Public Health*, 19(13), 7737.

Kaplan, D. M., Wade, M. E., Conteh, J. A., & Martz, E. T. (2011). Ethical framework for the use of social media by mental health professionals. *Counseling and Human Development*, 43, 12.

Kapoor, K. K., et al. (2018). Advances in social media research: Past, present and future. *Inf Syst Front*, 20, 531–558. doi:10.1007/s10796-017-9810-y.

Lehanot, K., et al. (2010). Psychotherapy, professional relationships and ethical considerations in the MySpace generation. *Professional Psychology: Research and Practice*, 41(2), 160–166.

Liu, C., et al. (2018). Using artificial intelligence (Watson for oncology) for treatment recommendations amongst Chinese patients with lung cancer: feasibility study. *Journal of Medical Internet Research*, 20, e11087. doi:10.2196/11087.

Miner, A., *et al.* (2018). Key considerations for incorporating conversational AI in psychotherapy. *Frontiers in Psychiatry*, 10. doi:10.3389/fpsyt.2019.00746.

Rein, B., *et al.* (2018). Evaluation of an avatar-based training program to promote suicide prevention awareness in a college setting. *Journal of American College Health*, 66, 401–411. doi:10.1080/07448481.1432626.

Steinberg, J., Beaver, K., Winkler, I., & Coombs, T. (2023). *Cybersecurity All-in-One for Dummies*. Chichester: Wiley.

Index